GW00322583

A textbook of
Aromatology—the science of essential oils for
the whole person
by
W. E. ARNOULD-TAYLOR

*Member Section Epidemiology
and Community Medicine —
Royal Society of Medicine*

Other books by the same author:

The Principles and Practice of Physical Therapy
A Textbook of Anatomy and Physiology
Ultrasound Treatments
Electrology: Theory and Practice

Phys-essential Therapy

Aromatherapy for the Whole Person

by

W. E. ARNOULD-TAYLOR
M.Sc., Ph.D.

Stanley Thornes (Publishers) Ltd

First published in 1981 for

Arnould-Taylor Education Ltd
James House, Oakelbrook Mill
NEWENT GL18 1HD

by

Stanley Thornes (Publishers) Ltd
Old Station Drive
Leckhampton
CHELTENHAM GL53 0DN

Reprinted 1984
Reprinted 1990
Reprinted 1991

British Library Cataloguing in Publication Data

Arnould-Taylor, W.E.
    Aromatherapy for the whole person.
    1. Aromatic compounds
    I. Title
    547',6   QD331

    ISBN 0 85950 337 2

Text set in 11/13 Century Old Style, by Buckway
Printing Co. Ltd., Cirencester.
Printed and bound in Great Britain at
The Bath Press, Avon.

CONTENTS

PART I

PART II   65

FOREWORD

This book started life in a more modest form several years ago as a science and therapy monograph published for private circulation by Arnould-Taylor Education Limited. Because of the extensive demand for the monograph from all parts of the world it was decided to update it and expand it into the form of a book. After consultation with some of my colleagues, I came to the conclusion that such a book would be much more useful if it contained a variety of experience. I therefore invited the co-operation of a number of people who use essential oils regularly in their practice to provide me with case histories, thus enabling the reader to see what can be achieved by the selective use of these oils. I would like to thank all the contributors for time and effort they spent in providing the information and detailing it in such a way that it could be copied by others, also Jane Cryer for her painstaking typing of the scripts, Mrs Rosemary Wise for the excellent botanical illustrations and Oxford Illustrators for the others.

I would particularly like to place on record thanks to my colleague, Mrs. Kim Aldridge, who, over the past 35 years, has done so very much not only to popularise the use of essential oils but to help an ever-increasing number of practitioners with the problems that they face from time to time. I would also like to thank her for reading the proofs and for her encouragement and constant prompting without which this book would not have been possible.

William Arnould-Taylor

Part I

Chapter 1

Introduction

The writer's association with essential oils started over 35 years ago through a friendship in Paris with Madame Marguerite Maury and her physician husband. At that time as a member of a World Scientific Committee of applied physiology, meeting at the United Nations Educational Headquarters in Avenue Kléber, Paris, frequent visits to the French capital were necessary. Marguerite Maury expressed a wish to establish her aromatherapy practice in the United Kingdom. Assisted by a well-known London physiotherapist, Ms. Taylor (no relation) and Miss Kim Solly, as she then was, a number of training seminars were organised and these together with the resultant publicity enabled Madame Maury with her protéges to commence her practices in Great Britain. Unfortunately, Madame Maury's sudden death prevented her from seeing the full success of her work, but her clients were very well looked after and her practice considerably expanded later in the form of two separate practices by her former assistants, Micheline Arcier and Danielle Ryman.

The early days for this new therapy were by no means easy. Very few people other than chemists had even heard of essential oils and even fewer had any idea of their potential. When any new idea is introduced in the field of health it is inevitably greeted with enthusiasm by a few, suspicion by some, scepticism by many; whilst the majority adopt an attitude of 'wait and see.' It is only necessary to read the lives of scientists like Pasteur and Marie Curie to realise that the reaction to aromatherapy was in no way unusual. However, some 25 years on, the position is materially different and the fairly frequent reference to aromatherapy in the recent past, on both radio and television, shows wide acceptance of this as a serious therapy: the word has cut a niche for itself in the English Language.

A good example of how the medical profession eventually accepts a new idea in other, and sometimes unorthodox fields when its value has been proved, is to be found in the case of ultrasonic treatments. The writer has been involved in ultrasound since 1948 when it was first introduced into Isleworth Hospital on an experimental basis. It was subsequently rejected as being unsuitable for use in the National Health System. During the next 10 years the use of ultrasound was limited to private clinics and osteopaths who were quick to recognise its therapeutic worth. As evidence of its value built up, the message gradually infiltrated the hospital system until the present time when almost every physiotherapy department has at least one ultrasound unit.

As with all therapies there are misconceptions, misunderstandings and sometimes perversions; the writer felt that it was necessary to clarify the science of essential oils as he sees it, and with this object in view the raison d'être for this book may be summarised: firstly, to place the science of essential oils in their proper perspective; secondly, to state clearly and simply the values as well as the limitations of essential oils; and thirdly, to encourage a scientific approach to a subject which is much more than usually susceptible to unscientific mumbo-jumbo. In this particular field of applied physiology, there is constant development and discovery, much of which is exciting. It is hoped that the following chapters will encourage many others to explore for themselves and so add to the sum total of knowledge and experience of essential oils.

:   *If you love something, set it free*
:   *If it comes back – it is yours*
:   *If it doesn't – it never really was*

Chapter 2

History

The history of the application of essential or aromatic oils to the human body must be almost as old as history itself – its beginnings being lost in antiquity. The oldest medical book of which we have knowledge was published in China some 2 000 years before Christ. It was written by the Emperor Kiwang-Ti. He refers to several essential oils whose properties he had recognised – these properties were basically the same as those of today. However, our first evidence of the wide use of aromatic oils comes from ancient Egypt where the priest doctors used aromatic oils and gums as burnt offerings to their gods. The preservative qualities of these oils were also well known to the Egyptians who used them extensively in embalming the dead and it is said that when archaeologists opened the tomb of Tutankhamun, the odour of kyphi, one of their favourite oils, came forth. The Assyrians are credited with being one of the first people to use essential oils more for sheer pleasure than for religious rituals. It is said that at the games at Daphne several hundred girls were employed to sprinkle spectators with oils from golden bowls. In fact it was the Babylonians' extensive use of essential oils that brought early prosperity to Southern Arabia – an area which held a strategic position on the trade routes from India. History records that it was an Arabian physician who first created a method of distilling the essence of flowers and for several thousands of years India was probably the greatest source of many of the Old World's favourite oils: cinnamon, spikenard and myrrh.

In the Old Testament we see in the songs of Solomon reference to the valuable sources of such oils: 'Thy plants are an orchard of pomegranates with pleasant fruits, camphire with spikenard, spikenard and saffron, calamus and cinnamon with all trees of

frankincense, myrrh and aloes'. In a press report emanating
from Cairo in March 1978: 'Archaeologists here claim to have
discovered the secret of Queen Nefertiti's legendary beauty. For
cleansing the pores of her skin she used facial beauty masks
made up of honey, milk and flower pollens and for keeping her
skin soft she used a potion of orchid leaves and honey and in her
bath went the oils of 80 different herbs and fruits'. In the Grecian
empire, which followed, medicine became the subject of more
serious and scientific study and in the days of Hippocrates the
medical uses of a number of essential oils were categorised. The
succeeding Roman empire capitalised on this knowledge and it is
reported that in the city of Capua an entire street was occupied
by essential oil manufacturers.

Some of the raw materials used in the industry at the time of the
Roman empire were so costly that slaves who worked in the
establishments were stripped and searched every night before
being allowed to return home. In another part of this book
reference is made to the high cost of essential oils today, so it will
be seen that things have not altered that much in 2 000 years.
Because of the high value placed on these oils it is perhaps not
surprising to find that when the Three Wise Men brought their
gifts to the infant Jesus, they brought with them the three most
valuable they knew – gold, frankincense and myrrh.

In the New Testament we find further reference to oil for healing
purposes when Christ tells the parable of the traveller who had
been set upon by thieves and left injured at the roadside. He was
seen by a Samaritan who rendered first aid by pouring oil and
wine into the wounds (in those days wine was extensively used as
an antiseptic). Following the decline of the Roman empire we
lose sight of essential oils until about the 13th century, though
this gap may only be caused by the almost complete absence of
any detailed records of that period. In the 13th century we learn
of distillation being applied to plants and flowers which
coincided with the achievements of the famous Bologna School
of Medicine by its contribution to anaesthesia of the *Spongia
soporifica*. It is more than likely that this anaesthetic originated
many years before in India but we are indebted to Hugo of
Lucca – whom some regard as the founder of Bologna Surgical
School – for the prescription of this anaesthetic. This was to soak
a sponge in an ounce of each of the juices of unripe mulberries,
flax, mandragora leaves, ivy, lettuce seed, lepathum and
hemlock, to which was added hyoscyamus in a brazen vessel.
The whole was then boiled and stored for use.

Reference has already been made to the pouring in of oil and wine into the wounds of the traveller. It is not surprising to note that the relator of this parable was St. Luke, the beloved physician, and he was simply telling what was currently accepted in his day. The very famous Greek physician, Galen, was a fervent believer in the efficacy of wine poured into a wound and it is on record that whilst he was medical officer to the Roman gladiators his method of treatment was so successful that not one gladiator so treated died of his wounds.

From the Bologna School of the 13th century and its famous sons, Hugo of Lucca, Theodorick of Servia and Paracelsus, until the 19th century there was continual use of essential oils in the treatment of disease. Today the centre of the world's essential oils industries can be found in Grasse, an ancient provincial walled town behind the French Côte d'Azur. It is interesting to note that its supremacy in this field originally came from the fact that it was an important leather-making centre. It was in the middle of the 16th century that Catharine d'Medici imported from Italy a fashion for scented gloves – a fashion which Grasse's businessmen were soon able to capitalise on because of the large quantities of lavender and herbs that grew in the French Alpine foothills. With the passage of time, the fashion for scented gloves died out (due in no small part to the prohibitive taxes which were placed on fine leathers) and the Gantier-Perfumeurs gave up leather making and concentrated on essential oils instead.

In this connection, it is interesting to note historians have related in Paris and London during the cholera epidemic that the glovers enjoyed an immunity from the plague which was denied to others. The English tradition of a posy of lavender and other herbs carried before an Assize judge dates from the time when these were the only antidotes known against the dreaded plague and it was their liberal use in the law courts which allowed justice to be continued. About this time, and for a long time afterwards, lavender was a highly respected means of protection against the 'vapours'. The scientific basis of antisepsis was not known at this time and it was commonly believed that disease was breathed into the body. Lavender was considered to be a good form of protection against many such diseases and became a very flourishing industry. Children were encouraged to wear lavender lockets, that is silk bags stuffed with lavender, around their necks and lavender sachets were liberally sprinkled amongst clothes both to keep them fresh and as a protection against moths and other insects. The pleasant fresh smell of lavender must also have been a very pleasant relief in those days against the accumulation of human and other smells. Royalty were amongst those who extensively used lavender and one is tempted to believe that it might have been necessary because the chronicler of Queen Elizabeth I records, 'Her Majesty took a bath every six months whether she needed it or not.'

In the 15th century the first *Eau Admirable* was created by J. M. Feminis. This led his nephew to manufacture the famous *Eau de Cologne MM Ferina* which later proved to be a reasonable antiseptic. During the 19th and 20th centuries however, the use of essential oils was eclipsed by the rapid discovery of new and synthetic substances, many of which were very effective but were not without side effects.

In the early part of the 20th century there was a slow but natural movement towards purer forms of treatment and with it came a rediscovery of the value of essential oils. Much of the credit for this rediscovery may reasonably be attributed to the famous chemist Professor R. H. Gattefosse. During the 1st World War the only antiseptic in common use was phenol, more commonly known as carbolic acid. This substance was reasonably suitable for swabbing hospital floors, but it was not a particularly good antiseptic for use on open wounds. In the first place, it was not very strong, secondly its side effects – notably those of acid – burning made it a less than perfect antiseptic. It was at this time that Dr. Gattefosse was able to conduct a lot of experiments on soldiers and found that it was possible to considerably accelerate the healing process of wounds using certain oils, notably lavender, which were able to penetrate the skin to the extra-cellular liquids which in their turn carried them to the blood and lymph systems which are an essential part of the healing process. It is recorded that during the experimentation in his laboratory, Dr. Gattefosse burned his hand and immediately plunged it into a container of lavender essence with the result that within a few hours the burn had disappeared. It is however, surprising to the writer that it took so long for the antiseptic qualities of lavender to be recognised because for some 200 years before this time oil of lavender had been used by the Swiss as an antidote against adder bites. Similar results to those of Professor Gattefosse are confirmed by the French physician, Dr. Jean Valnet in his book *Aromatherapie.*

A keen student of the work of Dr. Gattefosse was another biochemist, the late Marguerite Maury. She carried his work to a more practical conclusion by creating a number of well researched formulae which her physician husband was then able to use. Over a period of several years they were able to build up considerable experience of the effect of essential oils over a wide variety of disease conditions. Subsequently, Marguerite Maury spent a good deal of her time in teaching and right up to the time of her death trained many therapists in the special techniques which she had developed, and this large number of disciples has been largely responsible for the greatly increased interest during the past few years in the subject of aromatherapy.

Chapter 3

The Rationale of Essential Oil Treatments

A prayer for all therapists. 'From treating patients as cases and making the cure of disease more grievous than the endurance of same Good Lord deliver us.'

As mentioned in the previous chapter the 19th century and the first half of the 20th century witnessed the belief that chemotherapy would provide an answer to all the diseases to which man is heir. Whilst during this period tremendous strides were made in the field of preventative medicine, it must be observed that the high hopes entertained for many drugs have not been reflected in achievement and after much research and the expenditure of many millions of pounds such disease conditions as the common cold are still well and truly with us. An enlightened and educated society was not slow to appreciate the shortcomings and reflected that some of the older remedies and ideas might well be worth another try. The past 20 or 30 years have therefore seen a tremendous upsurge of interest in more natural products such as fresh fruit and vegetables, foods rich in fibre and a moving away from foods based on manufactured sugars. This general movement has not gone unnoticed by the medical profession and a report published in 1980 of a working party chaired by Sir Douglas Black, President of the Royal College of Physicians, echoes what health food pioneers have been saying for years. They say that too many people in Britain are eating the wrong food and that to avoid many diseases of Western civilisation, the British diet should contain more fibre.

At the same time, we find the Health Education Council (a Government-sponsored body) publishing a poster in which they say 'The doctor may not give you a prescription – his advice may be all you need. You can be sure that if you really need one you will get one.' In April 1978 a joint statement was made by David Ennals, the then Secretary of State for Social Services and Dr. James Cameron, Chairman of the Council of the British Medical Association, in which they say,

> The British Medical Association and the Health Departments share a growing anxiety about rising patient expectation and consumption of National Health Service facilities including pharmaceutical products and the implications these tendencies have for public health and Health Service resources. They recognise that the underlying causes of these phenomena are complex and attributable to diverse factors. Nevertheless, they ask every doctor to consider how best to contribute towards arresting the trend.

In this climate of growing awareness by the authorities of drug abuse and a movement towards more natural things we find essential oils providing an answer.

We live in an age when many people feel that an idea is not good unless it is complicated and the Englishman, who was once noted for calling a spade a spade, is now encouraged in Common Market parlance to think of it as a 'manually operated recreational eco unit maintenance tool.' The British publication *Motorboat and Yachting* recently reproduced an extract from a brochure for an Italian motor yacht, 'Simplicity not merely as simplification and reduction of the former range but at a programmed quintessentiality of the competence of the design vocabulary for throwing into relief the capacities of expression of the material.' The editor of *Motorboat and Yachting* commented, 'Fortunately, enclosed with the brochure is some actual information about the boat!' Further comment on the complexity with which we surround ourselves, Alwin Münchmeuer, a top German banker, is credited as having said, 'The Lord's Prayer has 54 words, the Ten Commandments 317 words but a Common Market directive on the import of caramel and caramel products goes to 26 911 words!'

The writer notes with regret that there has been a tendency for some people to extend this complexity to essential oil treatments in a way which is confusing and detracting from their original simplicity in use. Some people link essential oils treatment with astrology and a number of fringe medical ideas. Whilst the writer recognises that the people who believe in these ideas have every right to use essential oils in conjunction with them, he feels it weakens the role of essential oils as a therapy in their own right.

It should be emphasised that in no way should essential oils be used instead of ordinary medicine but rather supportive of it. Conditions still have to be diagnosed, and this should only be undertaken by persons whose training qualifies them to do so. It must also be noted that acute illnesses can often be best treated in an orthodox way. For example, at the onset of pneumonia there would be little justification for trying essential oils when certain antibiotics are known to be so effective, particularly as without the proper treatment the patient may well be dead in 5 days. On the other hand, the use of essential oils beforehand may well have prevented the onset of pneumonia.

The correct way to apply essential oils to the body is by massaging them into the skin, the reasons for which are given in a later chapter. The use of oral applications is to be deprecated. It is noted than in one of her lectures Madame Maury said,

> When we tried to administer by the digestive tract we found we had to employ essences which had been deterpenised owing to the sensitivity of the mucous membranes to pure essences and essential oils. This was a great disadvantage since we have found by experience that it is the very combined effect of terpentines and the trace elements which give aromatic substances their therapeutic value. On the other hand, we found that by effecting penetrations through the skin, diffusion was much more moderate and controllable. The dosage and the quantity absorbed was precise and we were able to control all the subsequent reactions.

Additionally, the essential oils may not be complementary to the medication being given by the patient's physician, and also the oils are materially altered when they come into contact with the chemical contents of the stomach especially the effect of the stomach's hydrochloric acid. For example, it is well known that cheese and shellfish which are perfectly natural substances can have very adverse effects when taken with certain medicaments. Also, yeast tablets, again a quite natural product, when taken with certain antidepressants can trigger off a fatal internal reaction and even a daily dose of liquid magnesia to cure indigestion, can prevent absorption of some prescribed antibiotics. However, when they are applied through the skin, these problems are obviated because the digestive system is bypassed.

Many people have confused essential oils with herbalism and this is very understandable because of their common root. But whilst their philosophy is similar, their physiology is very different. In herbalism, usually a large quantity of the distillation needs to be taken because of it comparative weakness. In essential oils, quantities used are very small because of the high concentration. Futhermore, in essential oils it is easier to control both the quantity and quality of the product as will be seen in a later chapter. However, the two sciences have very much in common and reference to such things as peppermint, eucalyptus and sage serves but to confirm that these plants may be used in two different ways. Anybody who wishes to further explore the links will find interesting reading in the *Reader's Digest Book of Herbs* and Nicholas Culpepper's *Complete Book of Herbs.*

In concluding this chapter, it is emphasised that essential oils provide a simple straightforward treatment and that there is little justification for the complexity with which some people would encompass it.

Chapter 4

Scientific Considerations

It must be admitted at the outset of this chapter that most of the evidence in favour of the use of essential oils is of an empirical nature. Some experimental work has been done and almost certainly, much more will be done in the future. However, until much more has been accomplished in this research field it is not possible to exactly formulate the scientific basis on which essential oils work. However, it is not necessary to become too depressed by this absence of scientific data because the end result of all medical work is to be found in the patient. If, as a result of any treatment the patient's symptoms disappear, he is healthier, stronger and more mentally alert, then it may reasonably be assumed that the treatment was a success, and there is abundant evidence that essential oils fulfil this criterion.

A corollary is to be found in a number of other natural products which for hundreds, even thousands of years, depended on results for their continuance but eventually received scientific recognition because of research discoveries.

For several thousands of years the Chinese have used acupuncture as a means of anaesthetising patients about to undergo surgical operations. For many years the West generally considered that such claims were highly exaggerated and that when it did actually happen it was due to psychological factors. Recent work however at St. Bartholomew's Hospital, London, has shown that acupuncture practised for this purpose releases endorphins in the same way that morphia does and the value of the latter is well known. We still do not know the exact mechanism involved in the release of the endorphins but we do now know that this use of acupuncture has a sound physiological basis.

Countries around the Mediterranean have used garlic for many years for its antiseptic qualities, but recent experimentation reveals that garlic contains two antibiotic elements – allicin and garlicene, both of which are very active against staphylococcal infections. In slightly colder countries the onion, a member of the same family has been widely used for the treatment of colds and other respiratory disorders. More recent scientific work has however indicated that these plants may play a very valuable part in the treatment of heart conditions.

When the writer was in India recently he shared an hotel with an International Cardiac Congress. At this Congress Dr. D. N. Dhawan, Head of the Pharmacology Division of the Central Drug Research Institute at Lucknow said that both onion and garlic played an important part in the treatment of a heart condition known as hyperlipidoemia (high cholesterol in the blood). Other research work done at the Royal Victoria Infirmary, Newcastle, was by another Indian doctor, Dr. I. Sudharkaran Menon, this latter research was triggered off by a chance remark by a Frenchman who said that in his country, horses developing blood clots in the legs are treated with a diet of garlic and onions. With the collaboration of three of his colleagues, Dr. Menon set in motion a research project involving 22 patients who were recovering from stomach ailments and who were not being treated with any drug which would interfere with the study. Because exercise can help to dissolve blood clots the patients were made to stay in bed. They were first starved and then given a carefully controlled series of mammoth breakfasts. One group was given a large fatty breakfast, the second group the same meal but with the addition of fried onions. On the second day the groups were reversed, whilst in the meantime, a smaller section of the sample were undergoing the same experiment only with boiled onions. Throughout the tests blood samples were taken from all the patients who were involved.

The blood contains a substance known as fibrinogen which has a natural ability to change into a solid material called fibrin. The fibrin is a finely meshed scaffolding on which blood clots build. The function of the fibrinogen is particularly noticeable when the blood comes into contact with air through a cut or wound. It has been known for a long time that a high level of fat in the blood increases the capacity for fibrinogen to turn into fibrin and so increases the risk of clotting or thrombosis, but the work of Dr. Menon showed that the patients who had eaten onions, boiled or fried, had an increased capacity to dissolve the fibrin. It might at this point be worth noting that our ancestors who stuffed fatty foods like pork and goose with onions were not in any way unscientific even though they did not understand the basis for their actions.

Users of essential oils may be encouraged by the scientific discoveries which have been made in the above two studies but even though comparatively little research work has been done with essential oils what has been done is encouraging. In one experiment to show how essential oils are absorbed into the blood stream through the skin, a small quantity of essential oil was rubbed into a guinea pig's head and half an hour later a post-mortem examination showed traces of the essential oil in the animal's kidneys showing that it had made a complete circuit of the animal's vascular system and had reached the eliminatory system.

Research work has been undertaken by Professor Rovesti in Italy and Professor Vernel in the U.S.S.R. Work undertaken by the Institute Pasteur in Paris is particularly interesting where they found that the micro-organisms of yellow fever were easily killed by essential oils, particularly lavender and sandalwood. In a further test of the action of essential oils upon organisms usually encountered in the air, certain bacteria were exposed to the emanations from essential oils for various periods. The results indicate that many of the bacteria were killed in less than an hour and in some cases after only a few minutes.

Other research work has been done by Professor Omeltschenski. He found that the bacillus of typhoid fever was killed in 45 minutes by oil of cinnamon and the bacillus of tuberculosis destroyed in 23 hours by oil of cinnamon and 12 hours by oil of lavender or oil of eucalyptus. Cuthbert Hall showed that the antiseptic properties of the essence of eucalyptus were more powerful than the main constituent eucalyptol. In the same way, generally, essential oils are in total more active than their main constituents.

Although tempting, it is usually unwise for a scientist to prognosticate the results of future research but the writer feels that many of the answers will be found in the body's immune system. In days long past when he was at college, the writer was taught very little about the endocrine gland that we know as the thymus: situated high up under the breast bone, it was thought to have something to do with sexual maturation, but because it starts shrinking quite early in life, its role was considered to be a diminishing one. Recently medicine has taken an increasing interest in T-lymphocytes, sometimes called T-cells, the T standing for thymus derived. The T-cells enter the blood and lymphoid tissue where they attack viruses and bacteria. Another form of lymphocyte is the B-lymphocytes, the B standing for bone marrow derived and sometimes called B-cells, which are able to move directly into the peripheral lymphoid tissue where they are able to produce antibody molecules that lock onto invaders and incapacitate them. However, to be really effective this double pronged complex system needs to be triggered off and it would appear that natural enzymes act as catalysts which in turn produce the molecular model for the locking-on process which in turn triggers off the immune response.

The branch of immunology which is particularly concerned with the body's antigen systems is a comparatively new one but its development is exciting. Already more than 3 000 antigen patterns have been isolated and in some ways these patterns can be likened to pieces of a jigsaw puzzle. When another piece fits exactly into the irregular edge the immune response is triggered off. It therefore seems reasonable to the writer that essential oils, because of their enzymatic nature, may well be found to provide this necessary catalytic action.

Chapter 5

Essential Oils

WHAT THEY ARE AND WHERE THEY COME FROM

Essential oils are the vital elements of plants. They are considered to be vegetable hormones and they are extracted from varying parts of the plant. As examples, sage oil is extracted from the plant's leaves, neroli from the orange blossom flowers, tangerine from the fruit, sandalwood from the wood and cinnamon from the bark. True essential oils are very expensive to produce because they are so labour-intensive. Essential oils appear in larger quantities in the leaves of plants than they do in the petals, it requiring some 400 kg of parsley or thyme to produce 1 kg of the essential oil. When we move to the essential oils extracted from petals we find that gargantuan quantities are involved. It takes approximately 2 000 kg of rose petals to produce 1 kg of the essential oil whilst it takes about 6 tonnes of orange blossoms to produce 1 kg of neroli.

It will be appreciated that the plants producing these flowers have to be tended, the flowers harvested by hand, transported to the nearest distillery which may be some considerable distance away and then subjected to the usual distillation processes. This means that essential oils can, under no circumstances, be produced cheaply—a fact reflected in current prices which can be as high as £6 000 sterling per kilo. Because of the cost of the real product there must inevitably be imitations and as the popularity of essential oils increases so do the pseudo-oils. The latter may take one of two forms: either they are synthesised products, that is they rely heavily on a chemically synthesised base, or a very small quantity of the essential oil being diluted in a

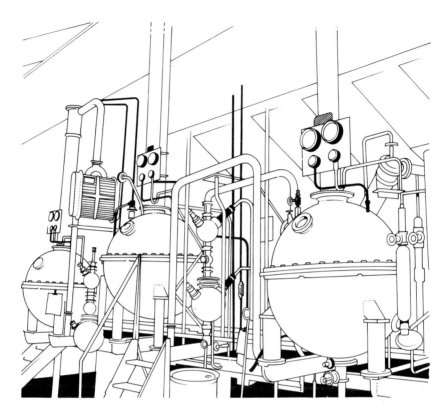

TYPICAL VIEW OF A COMMERCIAL DISTILLATION PLANT

spirit base. Because it is an odoriferous molecule it spreads itself very easily in alcohol. This is the primary method of producing perfumes and it takes an expert to really detect the difference between the genuine and the synthetic. It should also be noted that the quality of an essential oil is influenced by a number of factors, particularly its geographical and botanical source, the prevailing climate, the standards of local husbandry, the time of harvesting and subsequent treatment. The quality is almost invariably reflected in the price and as an example, Mediterranean jasmin, which is considered to be the best, is almost exactly twice the price of Egyptian jasmin, which is the one more generally used. Incidentally, the jasmin used in the products mentioned later on in this book is Mediterranean jasmin.

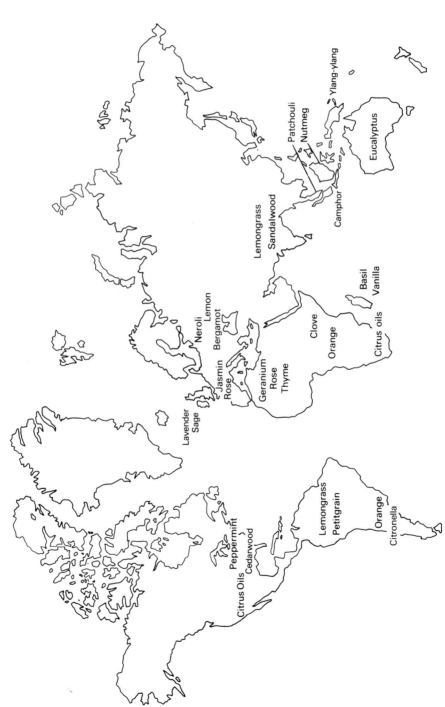

SOURCES OF SOME COMMON ESSENTIAL OILS

The town of Grasse in the South of France is now considered to be the headquarters of the essential oils industry but other countries do make their contribution to the sum total of the products. America produces a large quantity of peppermint and England has been famous for oil of sage for a very long time. History records that the first essential oil to be distilled on a large scale in the United Kingdom was sandalwood produced by Messrs. Stafford Allens in 1833 although it was not until 1885 that it found its way into the *British Pharmacopoeia*. The illustrative map accompanying this chapter will give the reader an indication of some of the main sources of essential oils, although it must not be taken as being comprehensive because there are many other areas that produce a variety of oils though usually in lesser quantities.

Essential oils are usually contained in oil cells in various parts of the plant and they can be seen under a microscope. They are generally colourless but there are some exceptions. Most essential oils are liquid but there are a few semi-solids such as araucaria, rose oil and wychwood oil which become liquid when heated to about 30°C. All essential oils are inflammable, very odoriferent and soluble in water and alcohol.

The orange tree provides an excellent example of how different oils are obtained from various parts of the plant. The rind of the fruit of the common orange yields orange oil – sweet orange oil from the sweet variety and bitter orange oil from the bitter variety. The blossom of the tree yields oil of neroli and the twigs produce a third oil – petitgrain oil. The presence of an essential oil can be demonstrated by igniting it with a match. There is one tree, the diptani, which grows in southern Europe, the leaves of which exude such a large amount of essential oil in hot weather that it can be ignited and in this way provide a natural fire hazard.

U.S.A.	Peppermint, Spearmint, Cedarwood
ENGLAND	Lavender, Peppermint, Sage
HOLLAND	Angelica, Caraway
GERMANY	Chamomile
BULGARIA	Otto of Rose
HUNGARY	Juniper Berry
SICILY	Citrus Oils

ITALY	Bergamot (it is interesting to note that the southern corner of Italy is the only part of the world where bergamot is produced commercially, although attempts have been made to produce it in other countries), Jasmin
SPAIN	Eucalyptus
RUSSIA	Coriander, Pine Needles
TURKEY	Rose
FRANCE	Lavender, Rose, Jasmin
ALGERIA	Geranium
PARAGUAY	Petitgrain
WEST INDIES	Lime
CHINA	Aniseed
INDIA	Sandalwood
SRI LANKA	Citronella, Cinnamon
SINGAPORE	Patchouli
EAST INDIES	Nutmeg
MANILA	Ylang-ylang
ZANZIBAR	Clove
EGYPT	Jasmin
AUSTRALIA	Sandalwood, Eucalyptus
PORTUGAL	Neroli

HOW THEY ARE PREPARED

There are five usual methods of preparation or extraction of essential oils. They are:

A. Distillation

D. Expression

B. Enfleurage

E. Solvent Extraction

C. Maceration

DISTILLATION

This is probably the oldest and most widely used method of separation of the essential oil from the plant. The process consists of heating the plant with water or with steam or both, in a still and channelling the vapour thus produced into a condenser. The liquid which results consists of a mixture of oil and water with the oil floating on the water or, as in the case of heavier oil—such as clove—the oil sinking to the bottom. It is then a comparatively easy matter to separate the oil from the water. Stills vary considerably in size, there are small ones used in the mountains by the small producer through to the larger ones which are carried on lorries and used particularly in the peppermint fields in the United States, or the very large ones evidenced in Grasse in France and Long Melford in England. The oils from the smaller distilleries are usually sold to a central buyer who is able to blend the various deliveries and, in this way, is able to offer a consistent quality.

DISTILLATION PLANT

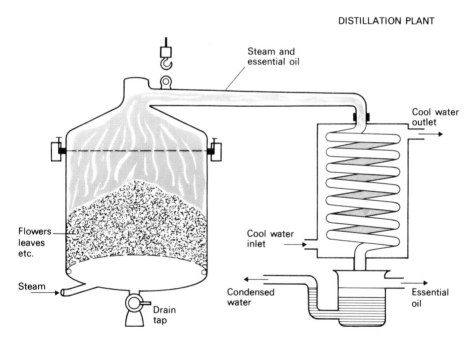

ENFLEURAGE

Both enfleurage and maceration depend on the physical fact that fat will absorb essential oils. The fat, of course, must be specially prepared because it has to be purified, odourless and unlikely to turn rancid. There are many recipes, often closely guarded by the families that own them, but most require a mixture of lard and beef suet. Enfleurage involves cold fat and is a method which may only be used for flowers which continue to generate essential oils after they have been harvested—jasmin being an example. A sheet of glass is mounted in a rectangular frame and a thin layer of fat is spread onto the glass. Onto this fat is spread a layer of freshly picked flowers. After about 24 hours the flowers will have given up all their oils to the fat. The frame is then turned upside down causing the withered flowers to fall off, another layer of freshly picked blosoms is strewn onto the fat and this process goes on for quite a long time—up to 70 days—depending on the flowers involved and the quality of the harvest.

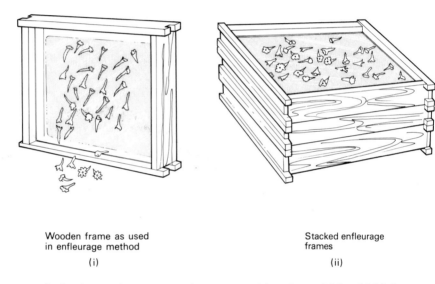

Wooden frame as used
in enfleurage method

(i)

Stacked enfleurage
frames

(ii)

A single workroom may house anything from 500—1000 frames. When the fat has been completely saturated with perfume it is then known as pomade: this is washed in alcohol whilst being mechanically agitated and in this way the essential oils are transferred to the alcohol. The alcohol is then evaporated leaving the essential oils.

MACERATION

This is a process which is applied to plants which do not generate essential oils after harvesting. The flowers are plunged into hot fat which penetrates the cells of the plants and absorbs their essential oils. The flowers are then removed either by centrifuge or straining and more fresh flowers introduced. This is repeated up to as many as 15 times and the resultant pomade is treated in exactly the same way as the product of enfleurage.

EXPRESSION

This process is reserved for the oils of the citrus family – lemon, orange, bergamot, grapefruit and tangerine. Up to about 1930 the oil was obtained by what has become known as the sponge process – the oil was extracted by being hand squeezed onto a sponge and when the sponge was saturated the oil was squeezed out of it. Skilled workers were able to exert just the right amount of pressure to obtain all the oil out of the rind but this was a rather costly process because of the labour involved so their work is now done by machine.

SOLVENT EXTRACTION

This is a process which may be applied to gums and resins as well as to flowers. With flowers the solvents used are usually either petroleum, ether or benzine, whilst in the case of resins and gums the solvent is usually acetone. The flowers or other base materials are placed in a vessel and covered with the solvent.

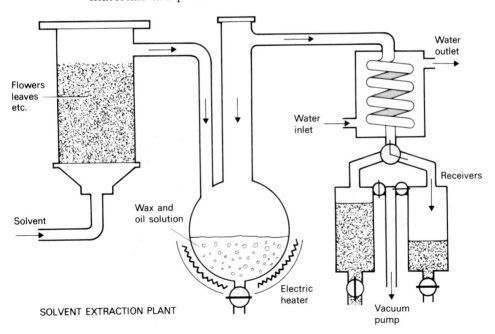

SOLVENT EXTRACTION PLANT

The mixture is then slowly heated – usually by electrical means, such as an electric flask blanket – during which process the solvent extracts the odoriferous principle of the material. This is then filtered resulting in a dark coloured paste which is known as concrete. This contains both the natural waxes and the odour-bearing matter. The concrete is then agitated with alcohol and chilled, the odoriferous constituents being transferred to the alcohol leaving the insoluble wax as a residue. The solution is then filtered and the alcohol evaporated off. In the case of resins and gums, these are dissolved by the acetone, liberating the active principles from the dirt and other insolubles. The solvent is then evaporated yielding a substance known as resinoid.

Chapter 6

Essential Oils – Their Uses

The uses ascribed to the various essential oils mentioned in this chapter are based on the assumption that they will be applied to the skin either in the form of a professional massage or at least with massage movements. Cutaneous absorption of the oil through the skin, subsequently into the blood stream when combined with therapeutic massage, is especially effective. The power of penetration is great; the time of absorption may be between 20 and 70 minutes. Some of the general effects of essential oils include encouraging the growth of new cells, delaying the process of ageing by eliminating the old cells more quickly, antibacterial action which in turn promotes healing, anticongestive action and the acceleration of toxic elimination. They help to relieve stress and tension by their effect on the peripheral nerve endings and, by increasing the elasticity of the skin, aid the reduction of scar tissue and stretchmarks. Used as general treatments they tend to create a state of euphoria and help to balance the physiological harmony which adds up to a sense of wellbeing both physically and mentally.

The uses associated with the following list of oils should be regarded purely as guidelines, in no way is it intended to override the judgement of the practitioner whose experience and knowledge of the patient will help him to decide which is the most appropriate oil for the condition being treated.However, for people who are new to essential oils or are in the early days of an aromatherapy practice, the list should prove a useful point of reference. It will be noted that a number of the oils overlap in their uses which gives the practitioner a good deal of latitude in choosing the most appropriate remedy. Also, because of this overlapping and the additional question of availability, some oils are more widely used in some countries than others.

The following list of oils, whilst by no means complete, is sufficiently comprehensive to indicate the wide variety of oils and the uses to which they may be put.

BASIL	There are something like 150 varieties of this in the world, the oil being obtained from the leaves, it has a tonic effect on nerves, is antiseptic and anti-spasm. Good for insomnia.
BERGAMOT	The oil is extracted from the pericarp of the fresh fruit, is antiseptic, a gastric stimulant and it is an essence often used in perfumery. Has a calming effect.
BENZOIN	Has a relaxing effect on the nervous system.
CAMPHOR (from Borneo)	Comes from Borneo and Sumatra and is obtained from the exudation of old trees. Was well known in Iran for its protective properties against the plague (not to be confused with camphor from Japan which is much cheaper and toxic).
CHAMOMILE	Is a gastric stimulant, tonic, anti-spasm, externally often used in cases of dermatitis.
CINNAMON	From the evergreen trees found in Sri Lanka, Java and Madagascar. The oil is obtained from the bark and the leaves, strongly antiseptic, haemostatic, and is reputed to be slightly aphrodisiac. Has been found to be very effective against scabies.
CLOVES	From a tree found in Madagascar and the West Indies. Anti-neuralgic, anti-spasm, antiseptic, slightly aphrodisiac. Well known for its analgesic effect on aching gums.

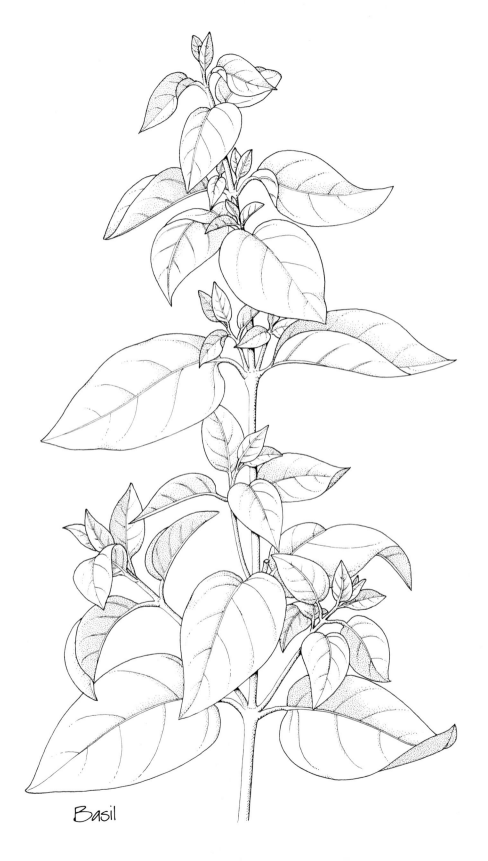

Basil

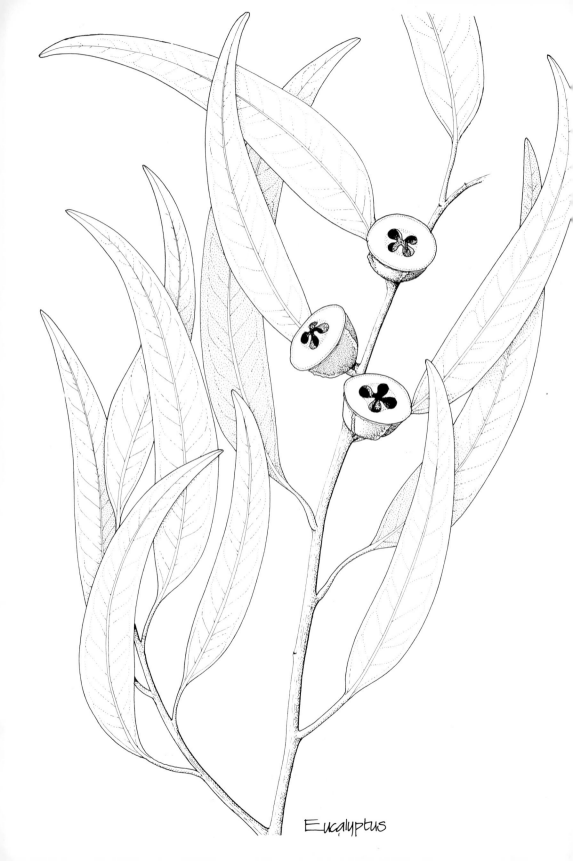

Eucalyptus

CYPRESS
The oil is extracted from the fruit. Has a vaso-constrictory effect on veins, is a diuretic and has been used effectively in menopausal upsets. A few drops at night on the pillow of a sufferer from whooping cough will help to check the coughing.

EUCALYPTUS
Originated in Australia but now found principally in the coastal regions of the Mediterranean. Well known for its use in inhalants for pulmonary conditions and for conditions affecting the sinus, nasal and bronchial passages. Externally it is useful for wounds and insect bites.

GALBANUM
An oil obtained from a plant which grows in Iran. Its properties are very powerful as a rejuvenating remedy. It should not be used in the treatment of young people.

GERANIUM
A plant of which there are some 700 species. Its principal effect is on the blood, helps to dissolve haematosis, making blood more fluid, having a general effect on circulation. Anticoagulant, useful on people with pale complexions. Useful as an astringent.

JASMIN
The essential oil is extracted from the flowers. Sedative action on nerves, tones the skin. Helps to prevent scarring, increases skin elasticity by its effect on the fibroblast cells.

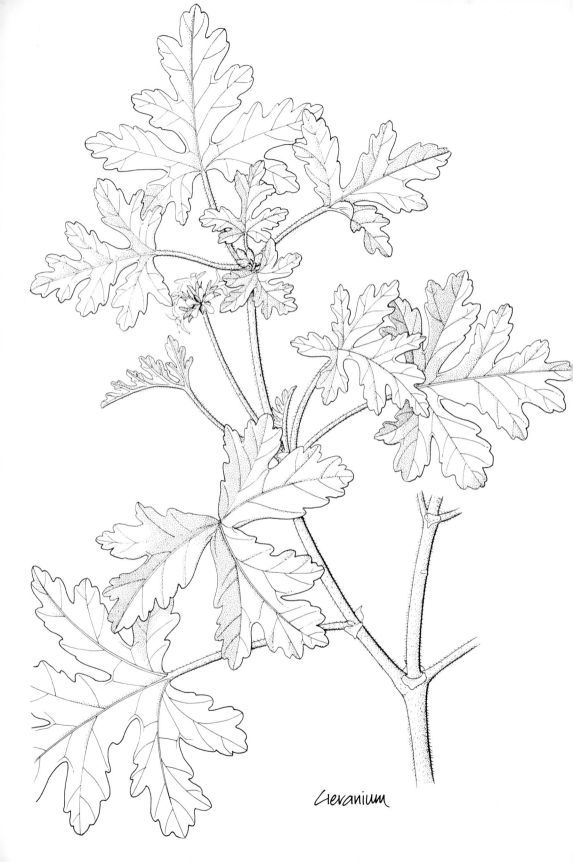

Geranium

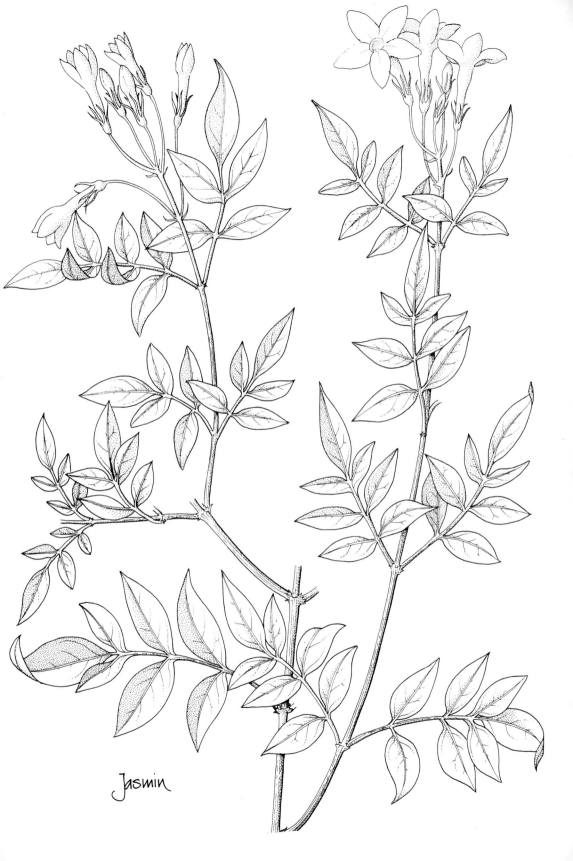

Jasmin

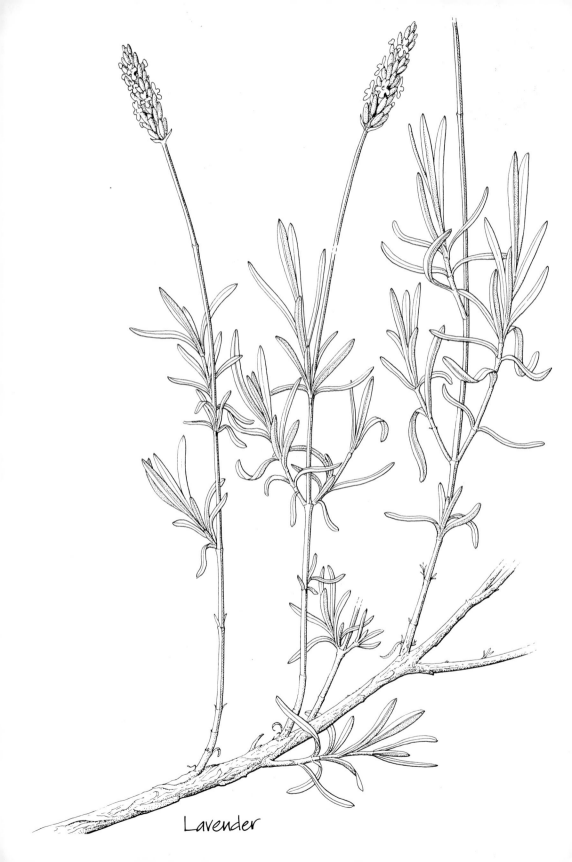

Lavender

LAVENDER	Antiseptic, very diuretic, anti-rheumatic, good regulator of the nervous system, very useful for use on wounds, burns, bites and some dermatitis. May be used on delicate or sensitive skins.
LEMONGRASS	Strong bactericidal effect, useful for treatments of skin with open pores and acne. Induces a revitalising process. Penetrates easily making muscles and skin supple and healthy, helps improve energy, builds up resistance to fatigue, very good on tired legs and venous conditions.
MARJORAM	Anti-spasm, calming, arterial-vasal dilator, useful in treatment of rheumatic conditions and nervous stress.
NEROLI	Extracted from orange blossom petals. Bactericidal, calming, improves skin elasticity.
PEPPER	Used in Greece for combating intermittent fever (a mild form of malaria). Improves muscle tone.
PEPPERMINT	Is well known for its decongestant effects, is cooling and anti-inflammatory which makes it very suitable for treating cases of sunburn whether caused by exposure to natural sunshine or acquired through sunbeds or exposure in solaria.
ROSE	Has many healing virtues, anti-bacteriological, aphrodisiac, a regulator of female functions, slightly astringent effect on the skin.

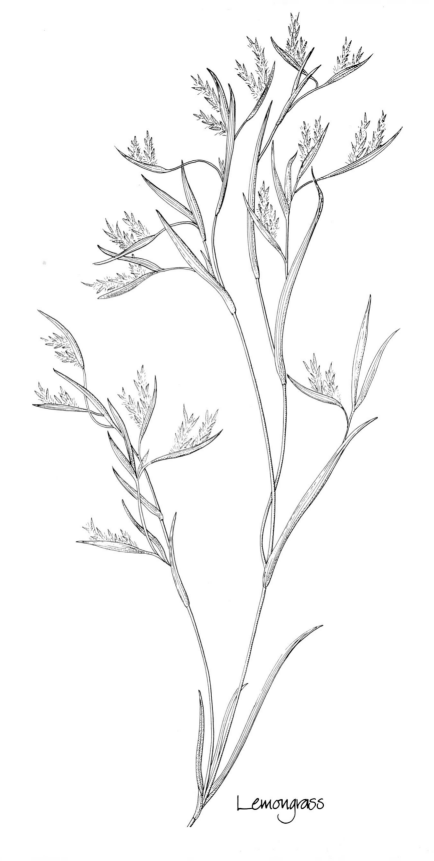

Lemongrass

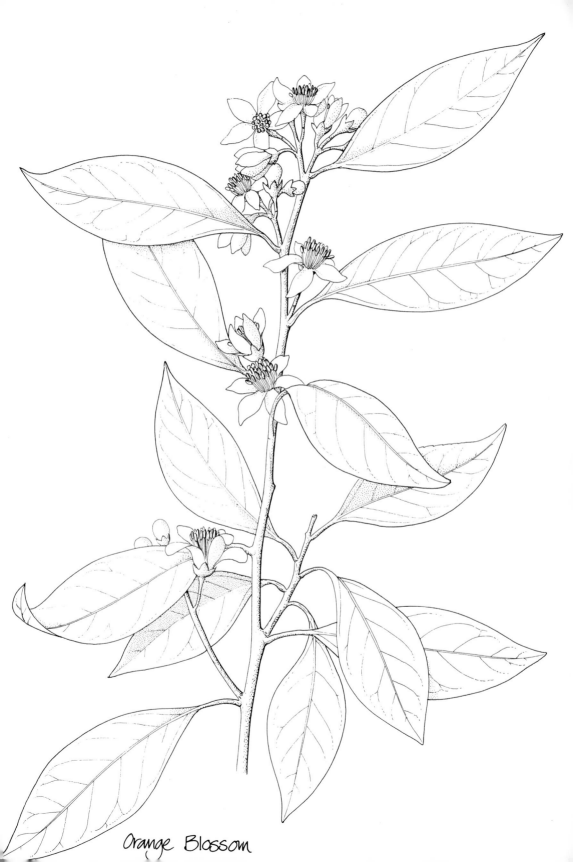

Orange Blossom

ROSEMARY   This essential oil is extracted from the flowers and leaves. Cardiac stimulant, anti-rheumatic, useful in treatments of obesity, especially where there is fluid retention.

SAGE   Grown the world over but some of the best is from England. Essential oil obtained from the flowers and leaves. Stimulant, antiseptic, diuretic, astringent, anti-fluid retention and because of its affinity for muscle fibres, is useful in cases of fibrositis, torticollis and aches and pains in over-exercised muscles. Suitable for all states of fatigue, particularly after strenuous effort.

SANDALWOOD   The essential oil is extracted from the wood. Has a strong antiseptic effect, for softening skin and the treatment of broken veins. Has a very relaxing effect.

STYRAX   Is a resin coming from a very old tree in Mexico and Central America, has a positive action on severe skin conditions and also acts as a rejuvenating agent.

TANGERINE   An oil particularly useful for the treatment of children and young people because of its tonic qualities and the way in which it improves the circulatory system, especially the peripheral circulation. Because of this latter property, it may be used effectively on people with pale complexions.

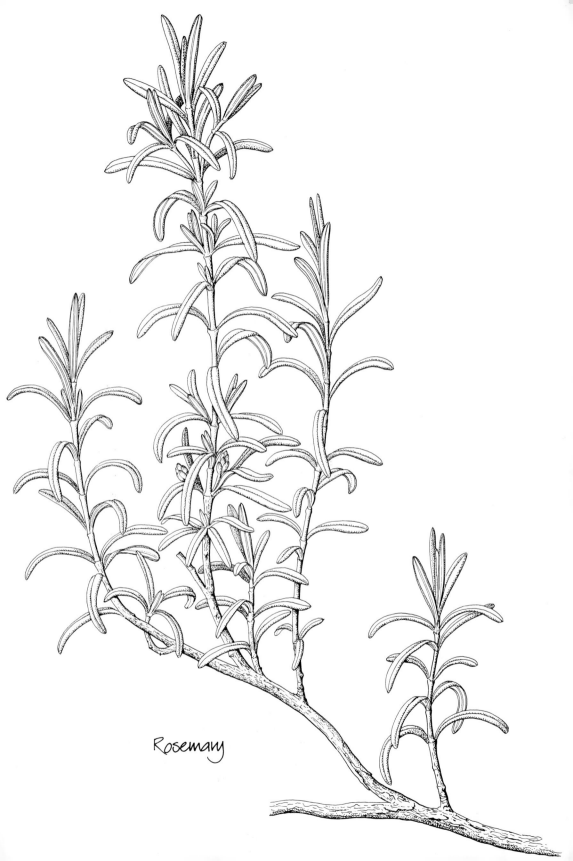

Rosemary

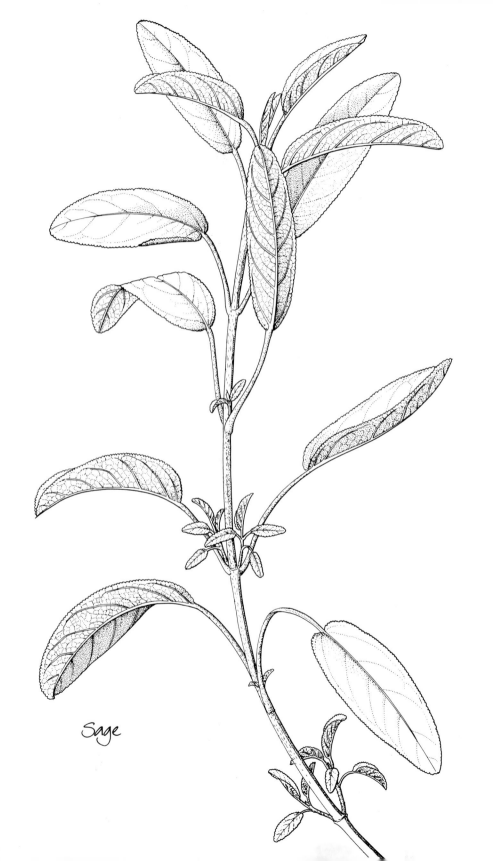

Sage

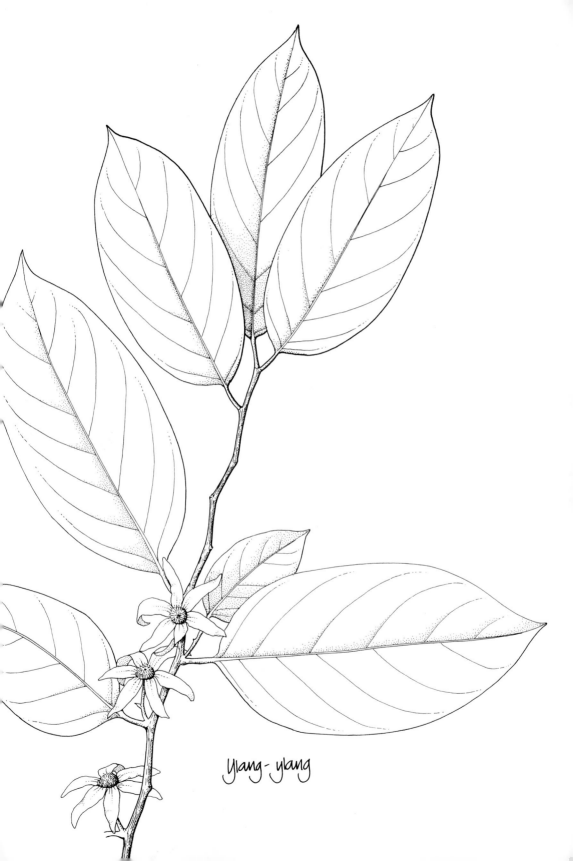

ylang-ylang

THUJA   *The tree of life* originally found
                           in China, now cultivated in
                           parts of France. It is an expec-
                           torant/sudorific   and   anti-
                           rheumatic. It is also useful in
                           the treatment of warts, polypi.

T H Y M E   Strong   general   stimulant,
                           antiseptic, aphrodisiac, useful
                           for some cases of dermatitis,
                           boils and carbuncles.

YLANG-YLANG   The essential oil being extrac-
                           ted from the flowers. Strongly
                           antiseptic, aphrodisiac, heart
                           regulator, useful in treatments
                           of impotency and frigidity.

In practice, generally, one or at the most two, oils are used on the
same patient. However, for some conditions a combination of
oils has been found to be desirable and these are made up to a
very carefully worked out formula. Their use is dealt with in the
treatment section.

Chapter 7

Essential Oils – Practical Considerations

Being the product of an orthodox education in physiology and chemistry the writer very naturally views with considerable concern the haphazard way in which essential oils are sometimes dispensed. As will have been seen from a previous chapter, essential oils are extremely concentrated which means that their formulation into a treatment mode should be very carefully controlled. To even approach the standard required by the *British Pharmacopoeia's* medications it is essential that the quantity (that is the formulation) be constant and the quality of a determined standard. In this chapter these two questions will be discussed separately because of their extreme importance to any practitioner seeking to achieve consistent repeatable therapeutic results without unwanted reactions.

QUANTITY CONTROL

The late Marguerite Maury, the bio-chemist who did so much to establish aromatherapy as a serious treatment, always dispensed her oils in two strengths; these were facial strength and body strength. This description is rather confusing until the basis on which it is founded is understood. As has been previously stated, these oils are dispensed for the purpose of introduction to the body through the skin, therefore, the formulation is based on the area of skin to be covered in the treatment. The more concentrated facial oils are designed not only for the face but for any area of the body approximately the same size as the face. For example, if the condition being treated was torticollis (wryneck) or lumbar fibrositis (lumbago), the area concerned would be approximately the size of a human face. On the other hand, body oils are formulated to cover a whole back *or* a whole front of a body. When the whole body is involved in treatment, a different oil should be used for the front from that used on the back – a point which is further elaborated in the treatment section. Essential oils themselves are too concentrated and too volatile to apply to the body in their pure form so it is necessary to blend them with a suitable base oil to give the necessary skin coverage.

These base oils must be of vegetable origin and should not become sticky under the action of the heat and pressure involved in massaging them into the body. These last two factors considerably limit the oils available for this purpose and in practice, cosmetic quality hazelnut oil and cosmetic quality soya bean oil have been found to be the most satisfactory. Avocado pear oil is a suitable medium when only a small area is to be treated, but it does tend to become rather sticky when massaged into a large area of the body. Madame Maury produced some very accurate formulations for the different oils in common use and these formulations were based not only on laboratory research but on treatment results on many thousands of patients. When a doctor gives a patient a prescription he knows the exact quantity of the active material which will be in the prescription. For example, if he advises the patient to take three aspirin tablets of 5 grains acetylsalicylic acid each four times a day, his treatment is being based on the absorption by the body of 60 grains of acetylsalicylic acid in a 24 hour period. If the quantity of acetylsalicylic acid in the tablets is not constant, varying say between 5 and 8 or 9 grains, this would mean that the patient would absorb a considerably increased quantity of acetylsalicylic acid and this instead of being helpful could in fact be deleterious because of the well known side effects of too much of this drug.

Accurate dosage in medicine has been the rule for very many years ever since it was demonstrated that whilst a little of the remedy may be very efficacious, too much of the same remedy could be harmful and in some cases, even fatal. However, many people seem to think that the same rule does not apply when the substances used are of a natural origin. Only a few years ago a man died in a Surrey hospital by eating too many carrots, the real cause of his demise being excessive vitamin A which is well known as being a cause of liver disorders and in children a loss of weight and hair. Another much flaunted vitamin, vitamin D, can lead to kidney stones and calcium deposits in the blood vessels when taken in excess. Such examples are in no way an argument against the use of vitamins A and D which are very essential elements for the maintenance of health in the body but purely to demonstrate that the body can have too much of a good thing.

Work-people handling the raw materials used in the production of some essential oils have to wear specially designed protective clothing to prevent their bodies absorbing any of the essential oils even in a very diffuse form. For example, work-people handling vanilla stocks tend to suffer from very bad headaches and intestinal upsets whilst extra heavy doses of saffron create convulsions and in some cases even death. Small quantities of marjoram are anti-spasm in action but large doses of it can paralyse which is the complete antithesis of anti-spasm, whilst digitalis, the essential oil of foxglove, which is widely used in the treatment of heart conditions can prove fatal if administered in too great a quantity. All these facts point to the necessity of an exact formulation if the body is to receive the full benefit of an essential oil treatment. The facts also demonstrate the inadvisability of people trying to mix their own oils unless they have received training in chemistry or pharmacy and at the same time have reliable formulae, because without such training it is very difficult to dispense accurately, because of the very small quantities involved in some of the formulations. Additionally, it is not sufficient to just mix the oils, they have to be blended, a point which all readers with the necessary background will readily appreciate.

QUALITY

This section can really be divided into two parts – the quality of the oils themselves and the factors which can alter that quality. First of all, oils must be brought from a reliable source where their quality is vouched for. The supplier mentioned at the end of this book buys most of his oils from Grasse and when there is a choice of country of origin, as a matter of policy he chooses the more expensive one, as evidenced in the case of jasmin where Mediterranean jasmin is purchased in preference to the much cheaper Egyptian variety. There are on the market some cheap oils but because of the very high price of the raw materials these cheaper varieties must of necessity be either diluted or synthetic, and it should be pointed out that it is not possible to accurately synthesise an essential oil. For example, analysis of the essential oil of rose has shown that it contains some 3 000 different ingredients, some only one part per million. On 19 April 1977 the British Broadcasting Corporation *Today* programme discussed oil of night primrose as a decoagulant treatment for coronary thrombosis and they pointed out in the programme that it was not possible to synthesise this oil because of 'some unknown factor'.

In Dr. Valnet's book *Aromatherapie* he tells the story of a patient who was suffering from an anal fistula which was being treated with natural lavender essence. The patient was almost cured when he had to undertake a business trip but forgot to take his essence with him, so he bought some at a chemist shop which unfortunately was neither pure nor natural and one treatment with this impure substance caused the poor man such a reaction that he was not able to sit down for 15 days!

Because of their susceptibility to ultraviolet light, oils should be purchased in amber coloured bottles. It has been observed that some oils are sold in clear glass bottles but no self-respecting chemist would allow this because he would be well aware of the chemical reaction caused by ultraviolet radiation and the subsequent alteration in the quality of the material. Essential oils should not be purchased in, nor decanted into, polythene or plastic containers (except for short periods for transit purposes), again because a chemical reaction will cause the oils to *go bad*. Finally, oils should be kept at an even temperature, that is neither too hot nor too cold.

Summarising this chapter, buy your oils from a reputable manufacturer rather than risk mixing your own unless you have the necessary training. Buy in amber bottles and if it is necessary to decant the oil then do so into coloured glass containers which do not transmit ultraviolet light and keep away from excessive heat or cold.

Chapter 8

The Use of Essential Oils in Body Treatments

Body treatments may be divided into two categories – general body treatments and specific treatments but before passing to descriptions of the two categories it is necessary to discuss a number of factors which are common to both.

Firstly, it is assumed that in these treatments the essential oils will be applied to the skin and then massaged in by hand. The skin therefore is our first concern. It is the largest organ of the body and acts as the barrier between the body's internal organs and its environment. It performs a number of functions but these may be narrowed down to the two principal ones – absorption and elimination. The very protective function of the skin makes its power of absorption limited to volatile

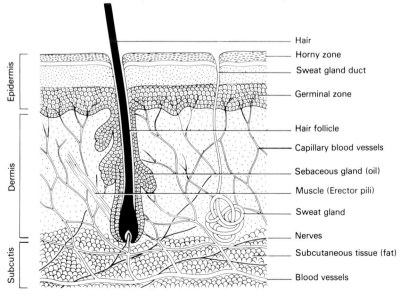

Epidermis

Dermis

Subcutis

Hair
Horny zone
Sweat gland duct
Germinal zone

Hair follicle
Capillary blood vessels
Sebaceous gland (oil)
Muscle (Erector pili)
Sweat gland
Nerves
Subcutaneous tissue (fat)
Blood vessels

THE SKIN

47

substances, for example, alcohol, certain vegetable oils and a number of medicaments including of course, essential oils. The eliminating function of the skin covers the giving off of excess body heat (the skin is the body's means of maintaining a constant internal temperature of 98.4°F) and getting rid of waste products and toxins as well as surplus body moisture.

Workers in hot countries where more of the skin is normally exposed can get rid of several pints of body moisture through the skin during the course of the day and in this way relieve pressure on the kidneys. In colder climates, the same kind of effect can be

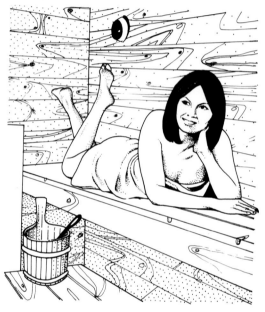

induced by the use of sauna baths and steam baths. These baths not only help the elimination process but also are a valuable aid to

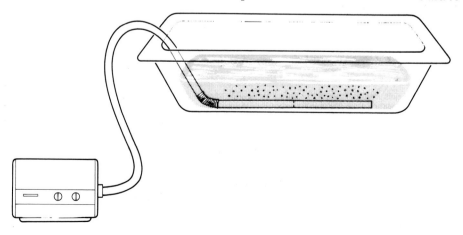

relaxation. However, it should be noted that when the body is eliminating it is not absorbing. So it is important that steam or sauna baths should not immediately precede an essential oils treatment. The eliminating process goes on for anything up to one hour after the sauna or steam bath has been terminated. It is therefore, advisable that the client should receive the bath treatments on another day or that there should be alternative treatments or a rest period in between the taking of the bath and essential oils treatment.

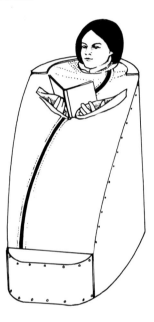

The odoriferous molecules of essential oils are vegetable hormones, living elements which are not destroyed by distillation or enfleurage but they are sensitive to heat and cold and germicidal action. If ray treatments are therefore to be

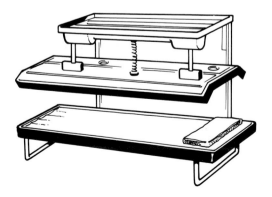

included they should precede the essential oils massage and never succeed it. Clients who are taking sunbed or solaria treatments can certainly benefit when these are followed by an essential oils treatment which will reduce, if not entirely eliminate, the dry itchy skin which so often follows exposure to ultraviolet rays.

Radiant heat (infrared) can play an important part in localised essential oils treatment. Amongst other things it dilates the pores and produces a hyperaemia by encouraging the blood into capillary circulation and in this way it helps the absorption and distribution of the oils.

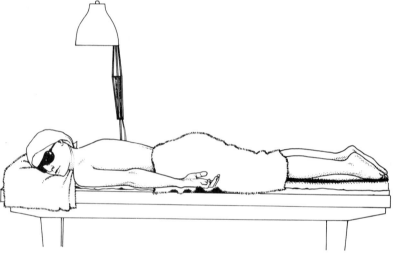

High frequency (sometimes wrongly referred to as violet rays) can also be a useful aid to treatment for small areas. The action of high frequency is to heat up subcutaneous tissue and to reduce tension on the skin surface, both of which actions encourage absorption of essential oils.

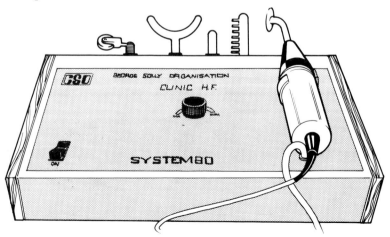

Practitioners who own an ultrasonic instrument will find this a very valuable tool for pushing the oils deeply into the body tissue. This process is known as phonophoresis and students who wish to pursue the study of this subject are referred to the writer's monograph on *Ultrasound Treatments.*

Full body massage with essential oils is normally performed for one of two purposes: either for its tonic, invigorating action or as a means of relaxation. Given for tonic purposes a useful guideline to follow is to use sage or jasmin on the back and lemongrass, lavender or rosemary on the front of the body. On the other hand, when the purpose is relaxation, sandalwood could be used on the back of the body and formula No. 2 on the front of the body. Such treatments will be spaced to suit the client's need and convenience but certainly should not be given more frequently than once in 24 hours and in most cases, less often would be preferable. In addition to full body massage, essential oils can play a valuable part in localised treatments and the following list gives some guidelines, although as previously mentioned, these should not be allowed to override the practitioner's experience and knowledge of the patient.

Respiratory problems – massage of the thoracic area with eucalyptus oil.

Epicondylitis, bursitis, synovitis – massage of the area and to the nearest practical lymph node with rosemary oil.

X-ray and other burn scars and stretchmarks – jasmin oil (or geranium oil if there is any suggestion of undue redness in the area).

Athletic stiffness, fibrositis – sage oil.

Cold extremities, chilblains and other circulatory problems – geranium oil.

Neurological problems – including neuritis, neuralgia and general nerve pains – basil oil.

Crêpy or saggy skin – (often seen after the client has undertaken a crash slimming course and especially evident on the inner aspects of upper thigh, inner aspects of upper arm and the bust region), muscle fatigue or debilitation – lemongrass, lavender or sage oil.

Localised slimming treatments – rosemary oil.

Cramp – when produced by cold or physical effort – sage oil. When organic origin – geranium oil.

Sports conditions – (too much squash, golf, tennis, etc. played infrequently) – sage oil.

Torticollis (wryneck) – treatment with sage oil, it is important to massage both sternocleidomastoid muscles because of their synergistic/antagonistic relationship.

Amounts used are quite small being approximately one teaspoonful of essential oil product to cover either the front or the back of the body or a coffeespoonful for specialised treatments, those which are treated locally.

In most of the above conditions, use of radiant heat or high frequency can be a very valuable adjunct to treatment. In the case of radiant heat the area to be treated should be exposed to the rays for about 10 minutes at a distance from the lamp where the skin is comfortably warm but not hot. Massaging with the oil should follow immediately the radiant heat is switched off, and at the end of the treatment it is important to make sure that the part is kept warm and free from draughts. Where high frequency is used as an aid to treatment the area should be covered with the mushroom electrode in small overlapping circles or with latitudinal strokes when the roller or curved electrodes are used. In the case of radiant heat it is essential to ensure that no oil or grease is on the skin before irradiation whilst in the case of high frequency it is usual to smear a little of the essential oil to be used on the skin as a lubricant before treatment and then the bulk of the oil will be used for the massage immediately afterwards. Where neither of the above instruments are available a reasonable alternative is the use of a friction glove which also has the hyperaemia effect.

The final consideration involving treatments is to prevent any oil that remains on the skin getting onto the patient's clothing with the consequent inconvenience to the patient and wastage of a valuable oil. To obviate this problem it is usual to use a good body milk to act as a sealer (i.e. form a film over the oil) which in turn encourages skin absorption. A product known as aromatherapy milk is particularly useful for this purpose because in addition to the usual skin milk qualities it includes essential oil.

To summarise this chapter, sauna or steam baths are useful for their decongestant, eliminatory action providing they are taken at least one hour before essential oils treatment. Full body massage may be given with the appropriate oils for either invigorating or relaxing purposes. In the case of invigorating massage the movements are invariably faster than those employed in relaxation massage. Radiant heat and high frequency can play a useful role in the heating of the area for specific treatments. Aromatherapy milk provides a fitting conclusion to the treatment.

Chapter 9

The Use of Essential Oils in Beauty Treatments

The author, not being an aestheticienne, is indebted to Mrs. Peggy Slight for her help in compiling the notes in this chapter. Mrs. Slight is one of the best known beauty editors of today and was amongst the first of Madame Marguerite Maury's pupils when she commenced training students in the United Kingdom. Beauty is inevitably related to the problem of ageing. Whether we like it or not, ageing commences at quite an early age. Certainly by the age of 23—25 the process of ageing has begun. Very obviously, this growing old of the skin cannot be stopped but it can be slowed down. To slow down the ageing process of the skin it would appear that three things are necessary:

A   Internal health, because the skin reflects the health of the body and most people would agree that if you are healthy you look healthy.

B   The skin must be decongested and kept as free as possible from the effects of air pollution, only too common especially in our large cities.

C   The treatment of the skin with substances which help to quickly eliminate dead cells and rejuvenate living ones.

A suitable method of facial routine for an aromatherapy treatment could run as follows:

1   Cleanse the face thoroughly. Madame Maury advocated use of a pulveriser such as the Lucas (sometimes referred to as Holo Electron). As has been indicated elsewhere in this book, steam causes the skin to eliminate and when it is eliminating it is unable to absorb. This means that facial saunas or hot steam applicators should not be used in aromatherapy treatments. However, the Lucas produces cool steam, that is steam which has cold water

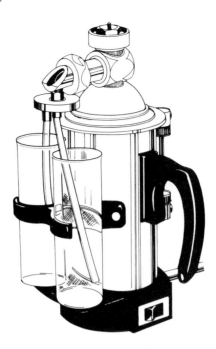

mixed with it by a process of capillary attraction from a separate container. This has the cleansing action of steam but does not cause the skin to sweat. If a cleanser is used on the face it should be cleansing milk and not cleansing cream.

2   Radiant heat may be applied to the face for up to 10 minutes in which case it is important to ensure that the client is not wearing contact lenses and it is advisable to cover the eyes with cotton wool pads. Alternatively, high frequency may be used on the face with the small size facial or mushroom electrode inscribing small overlapping circles and taking between 5 and 10 minutes to cover both sides of the face.

3   Following the diagrams (the original sketches for which were provided by Mrs. Slight) a thorough facial massage is undertaken using the oils which have previously been decided upon.

4   A cactus mask is applied very thinly over the whole of the face excluding the eyes. This, by forming a skin, will help force the oils more deeply into the tissue. After exactly 10 minutes the mask is washed off with a warm damp facial sponge. A special aromatic skin product such as Neroli Arome or Neroli Blossom may then be applied to the skin. This will act as a combined moisturiser and foundation. Heavy make-up should be avoided but a light dusting of powder is permissable.

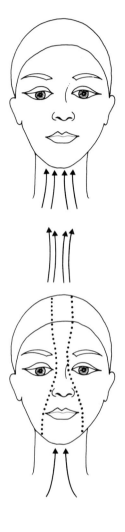

USING THE PRESCRIBED OIL

1.   Hold right hand for two or three seconds on diaphragm and perform gentle effleurage with alternate hands up to jaw line.

      As with all facial movements an even rhythm must be maintained.

2.   Firm pressures up the naso-mental lines using the second and third fingertips of both hands simultaneously.

      Without removing hands continue pressures up sides of nose to inner eye corner. Continue pressures up frontalis and back over epicranius to crown.

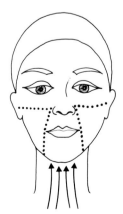

3.   Firm pressures up the naso-mental line using second and third fingertips of both hands simultaneously.

      Without removing hands continue pressures outwards along the antrum to the ear.

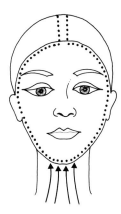

4.   Pressures from centre of chin up and around the contours of the face to centre of forehead and over epicranius to crown.

As with previous pressure movements using second and third fingertips of both hands simultaneously.

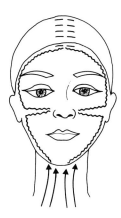

5.   a] With thumbs drawn outwards, splayed stroking descending from crown to hairline.

        b] Gentle vibrations along the path of the facial nerve. Vibrations are achieved by muscular contraction followed rapidly by relaxation which results in a fine trembling of the fingertips.

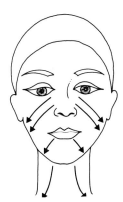

6.   Conclude with massage in a downward direction to increase lymphatic drainage by accelerating the lymph flow to help particularly elimination of waste matter.

After the body routine has been concluded return to the face and apply a Cactus Jelly Mask.

One big advantage of this type of facial is the immediate effect which it has – ageing skin looks younger, grey skin loses its ashen look and the texture becomes more soft and velvety. However, the maintenance of this condition raises a problem. In order to have a build up effect it is necessary for treatments to be given at least twice a week for five or six weeks and this, for reasons of time availability of the client, distances and economic considerations, is often not possible. In the circumstances the client should be encouraged to undertake home treatment in between the salon ones. Last thing at night the face should be thoroughly cleansed either with a cleansing milk or washed thoroughly with a good liquid soap, then using the bare fingers, a small quantity of the same facial oil as was applied in the salon should be thoroughly rubbed into the skin. Alternatively, as most clients are more used to using creams than oil, Neroli Cream makes a very good substitute. It should of course be left on all night and in the morning after following the usual cleansing process the cream should be replaced by Neroli Arome (or Blossom for younger clients), before applying light make-up.

Clients who are used to applying masks may like to use the cactus mask technique in which case they should be shown how to apply the mask last thing at night after having massaged the oil well into the face, the mask being removed after 10 minutes with a warm sponge as was done in the salon. Favourite oils for the face are jasmin for general purposes, lavender or lemongrass when a slight lift is needed, geranium when the skin is pale and anaemic looking, and rosemary when the skin has a puffy look caused by water retention. Acne condition is best treated with ylang-ylang oil but because of the extractive qualities of this oil it should be pointed out to the client that for a short while the condition may appear to worsen. This however, is a very necessary part of the process of draining the skin of excess sebum etc. and will only last for a short while. Do not use a mask with ylang-ylang treatment.

Because some clients, especially those visiting or living in warm/hot climates, tend to wear low-cut frocks or gowns it is worth noting that the facial type treatment including the mask can effectively be extended to include the decolletage.

Whilst on the subject of beauty, it is worthwhile noting that oil of rosemary makes an excellent tonic for the hair – being advisable to massage it well into the scalp after shampooing.

The substances used being natural ones, the question of allergies rarely arises. Should an allergic reaction occur, this can usually be overcome by substituting the particular oil used by another one in the same range. For example, if lavender has been used then lemongrass can be the substitute whilst if jasmin was used, geranium could be the substitute.

To conclude this chapter it is only necessary to indicate the respective uses of the different cactus masks. It should be noted that these masks are made from pure crushed cactus with the addition of essential oils. No other ingredients or preservatives being added. Geranium mask is normally used for pale skins as well as normal and strong texture skins. Lavender is used for oily skins, acne and where a facial lift is desired. It is also germicidal, so can be used wherever the skin is blemished. Sandalwood is used for sensitive skins, broken veins, diffused redness or wherever a relaxing facial is indicated. Jasmin cactus masks are useful for normal or ageing skins and wherever increased elasticity is required.

Chapter 10

Phys-essential Therapy

Phys-essential therapy is really an abbreviation of physical essential oils therapy. The therapists who practise this are people with rather special qualifications and with a motivation to help people with more serious problems than those normally encountered by the aromatherapist. There is a widespread belief amongst the public that aromatherapy is only related to beauty treatments. Whilst this is a mistaken belief, it nevertheless is so universally held that a number of therapists working in the more serious fields involved with essential oils and treating the whole person and not just the face felt that they should be recognised by a different name and so phys-essential therapy was born.

To qualify for this register, the person must first of all have undertaken the necessary training in anatomy and physiology and massage and hold a certificate such as the I.T.E.C. (International Therapy Examination Council) one, acceptable to local authorities for licensing purposes. Then they must have undertaken approved specialist training in aromatherapy and hold a recognised diploma in this subject. Finally, they must have undertaken the specialised training required for phys-essential therapy and hold the postgraduate diploma which enables them to state in their professional literature that they are a phys-essential therapist and are therefore entitled to use the letters Phys. E.Th. after their names. Not every aromatherapist wishes, nor indeed is suitable, to practise in this field because, in addition to expertise, it requires an understanding, sympathetic and patient personality. Above all, they must have the right touch. They are bound by the usual para-medical code that they only treat patients within the limitations of their own expertise and that they only treat medical conditions in co-operation with the patient's own physician. Whilst of course they are qualified to treat all those ordinary conditions which normally come within the purview of an aromatherapist they can, in addition, undertake the treatment of more serious stress and tension conditions, especially those arising from emotional causes.

The medical profession recognises that the one big killer of today is heart disease and it is estimated that currently one half of all deaths in the Western world are caused by this single but complex disease. Whilst there is not one precipitating cause, there is general agreement amongst the experts that at least a large part is played by stress, particularly the form of stress created by the patient having to face a set of circumstances over which he feels he has no control. The sad thing about this form of death is that it is hitting younger and younger people. In a comparatively few years incidences have changed from the 60—70 age group to be found frequently in the 30—40 age group and even in the 20—30 age group. In business it is to be found more often in executives on the way up, rather than those that have arrived, but it is equally associated with a mental inability to cope whether it be at work, following a bereavement or in personal relationships. Quite often such people develop a workaholic habit and always an inability to relax, though they are often the last people to recognise this fact.

Phys-essential therapists in addition to being good listeners (very essential in the early stages of the treatment) are supportive in their attitudes and use a number of relaxing aids to help accelerate the patient's complete recovery, at the same time fostering a healthy attitude to life so as to prevent a recurrence of the problem. Such aids may include a tape system to help relaxation on a daily basis, the use of suitable background music, advice an eating patterns, the necessity of regular but controlled exercise including underwater massage.

The special forms of massage which phys-essential therapists use involve the body as a whole and the long-ranging strokes employed provide the patient with a sense of whole body involvement rather than part treatment which usually happens in massage. Whilst neuro-muscular massage on the back is particularly aimed at the central nervous system, special emphasis is placed on massage at the front of the body and is directed at the sympathetic nervous system.

The writer having made a fairly intensive study of relaxation techniques came to the conclusion that the majority of them have one thing in common, that is, that they have to be learnt and this learning in itself is another workload to add to persons many of whom are not in a psychological condition to cope. Whilst therefore, yoga, transcendental meditation, etc. are very useful aids for those people who have the time and motivation to practise them, the writer felt that for seriously stressed persons what was needed was a series of commands which they simply had to follow and which required no forward thinking on their behalf and so avoiding another cause of stress. These command exercises last about 10 minutes and are followed by some associative treatment in the therapist's own voice so that the patient is mentally linked to his normal treatment situation. The advantage of this form of relaxation is that it may be undertaken almost anywhere – at home, or in an hotel room – and with the aid of a pair of headphones, even in a room where other persons are engaged in different activities. This is an aid which phys-essential therapists are using with ever-increasing success.

They also use an oil which has been specially created for the purpose. It consists of a blend of oils designed to effect the skeletal, muscular, central nervous, and sympathetic nervous systems. It is known as Formula 3 and it differs from the oils normally used in that one oil may be used for the whole of the body, back and front.

In concluding this chapter a phys-essential therapist's prayer might well be a paraphrased version of a well known one, 'God grant me the ability to help my patients to a mental attitude of serenity to accept things they cannot change, courage to change the things they can and wisdom to know the difference.'

Chapter 11

Conclusion

Anyone who has read the preceding chapters can hardly have escaped the conclusion that essential oils treatment is not only aimed at correcting deficiencies in the body's physiological process but is also an expression of a philosophical attitude to health and disease. It is in fact a reversal of the old doctor/patient relationship where the patient approached the doctor with, 'I am ill – make me better' and substituting for it the much more positive attitude of 'I wish to be well – teach me how'. Medicine has for too long spent a disproportionate amount of its time and resources in seeking the cure for disease rather than the promotion of health, but fortunately, those times would appear to be changing. In his book *The Political Economy of Illness* J. B. McKinlay quotes a story by Irvine Zola in which a doctor tries to explain the problems involved in the practice of medicine,

> 'You know,' he said, 'sometimes, it feels like this, there I am standing by the shore of a swiftly flowing river, I hear the cry of a drowning man. So I jump into the river, put my arms around him, pull him to shore, apply artificial respiration. Just when he begins to breathe there is another cry for help. So I jump into the river, reach him, pull him to shore, apply artificial respiration and then just as he begins to breathe, another cry for help. So back into the river again, reaching, pulling, applying breathing and then another yell. Again and again without end goes the sequence. You know, I am so busy jumping in, pulling them to shore, applying artificial respiration that I have no time to see who the hell is upstream pushing them all in.'

Essential oil treatments not only help towards the maintenance and improvement of health but encourages a new zest for living. The first principle, therefore, of any life extension programme is that health is a means to an end to enable a person to enjoy life for its own sake. The French philosopher, Jean-Jacques Rousseau its own sake. The French philosopher, Jean-Jacques Rousseau put it succinctly, 'Teach him to live rather than to avoid death. Life is not breath but action, the use of our senses, mind, faculties, every part of ourselves which makes us conscious of our being.' Put another way, to enjoy life is one of the best ways to lengthen it.

Into this new philosophy of positive health, essential oils fit very simply. They are natural substances tried and proved over the years and now combined with techniques which have been found to be very advantageous as a means of combating the several degenerative processes always in operation when the wellbeing and health of the human being is threatened. These natural substances have a very strong influence on the interchange of tissue fluids. They increase muscular and nervous tone, raise the general body resistance and make possible greater mental and physical effort. They favour cellular division and the creation of new and stronger cells which in turn influence the quicker and more efficient elimination of dead or worn-out cells. In this way toxic deposits and tissue debris are prevented from infiltrating the connective tissues which in turn achieves an improved tissue state – both in the muscle and the skin – which it is difficult to achieve by any other means. The mounting evidence of the efficaciousness of essential oils is based partly on scientific knowledge and partly on empiricism. Much work still has to be done to bring these two closer together and so overcome the air of mystery and sometimes downright scepticism of the part which may be played by aromatic substances in the attainment of a high degree of physical and mental health equilibrium.

Part II

Chapter 12

By Definition

The case histories which form this part of the book were provided by therapists who, in addition to their basic qualifications to practise, have taken postgraduate training in essential oils treatment. A number of them are members of the Phys-Essential Therapists Register; all are experienced practitioners (most of a number of years standing). So that the histories may be judged on their own merit, all therapists concerned have had their university or para-medical qualifications omitted. All the oils involved are to be found in the list in the appendix to this book.

To make this section easier to follow, the histories have been put under the most appropriate headings though this inevitably means a certain amount of overlapping. Some will not rightly fit into any of the enumerated categories and these have been grouped under *Miscellaneous*. In order to make reading easier, as well as facilitating cross-reference, the same format has been used throughout. In some cases the original report has had to be summarised but hopefully no essential information has suffered because of this.

It will be noted that in some cases the results were unexpected, in a number of cases the condition had proved resistant to other treatment, but in all the end result was satisfactory both to the therapist and to the patient.

These cases have been selected for their general interest because they cover a fairly wide range of conditions. During this particular research no deleterious effects were recorded and unwanted side effects were noticeably absent.

Chapter 13

Skeletal/Muscular Case Histories

Therapist: Sarah Charles, Cheltenham.
Sex of patient: Male.
Approximate age: 55—60.
Background information: Business man, executive status, travels extensively by car, driving himself, often involving very long journeys.
Condition treated: Lower back pain. Primary cause – client carried his lawnmower resulting in pain in the lumbar region. His doctor agreed to him having treatment which was commenced the same day.
Oil used: Sage.
Frequency of treatment: 2 days following, that is three days in all. On the first day it was virtually impossible for him to bend his back, on the third day he declared himself completely cured and drove himself to Wales. During the treatment, radiant heat was used on the patient before the oil massaged into the skin.
Result: Subsequent check-up recorded no return of the trouble although on a later occasion he had a similar type of problem with his arm making driving a painful proposition. He was given the same treatment, once only, and there was no return of the problem.
Comment: The only comment in this case came from the doctor who was very pleased with the result.

★ ★ ★

Therapist: Joy Sears, Leighton Buzzard.
Sex of patient: Male.
Approximate age: 30.

Background information: Warehouse manager.
Condition treated: Pain in lumbar region resulting from lifting a sack of potatoes.
Oil used: Sage.
Frequency of treatment: Once daily with radiant heat before the massage.
Result: Complete freedom from pain and work resumed in 48 hours.
Comment: The patient felt relief as early as half an hour after treatment.

The above therapist recorded an almost identical case history of a company director aged 30 who suffered small back pain as a result of carrying a filled oil radiator up a flight of stairs. Treatment was similar, that is radiant heat first followed by sage oil massage. A quarter of an hour's rest on the couch to allow absorption of the oil and 48 hours later reported that all pain had disappeared. Neither of the two patients reported any return of the trouble.

★   ★   ★

Therapist: Elizabeth Jane Guyett, Windsor.
Sex of patient: Female.
Approximate age: 40.
Background information: Housewife, kyphosis of spine and had considerable hospital treatment in the physiotherapy department but had learned to live with back pain.
Condition treated: Myalgia and stress.
Oils used: Sage on the back and No. 2 or sandalwood on the front of the body.
Frequency of treatment: Weekly with radiant heat being used before neuro-massage.
Result: After 2 months is free of back pain, feels confident, much more in control of herself. Treatment benefited both herself and her family.
Comment: By the therapist – 'I was surprised at the speed with which the treatment worked because I had estimated that it might take up to 6 months.'

The above therapist also records a case of a male patient aged about 32 who was an accountant in business on his own account having very little exercise other than weekend squash. In this case the condition treated was myalgia and fatigue and the oil used was sage with radiant heat as before. In this case the patient declared himself well pleased with the treatment as he is without pain and completely without stiffness.

★   ★   ★

Therapist: Jenny Hemingway, London.
Sex of patient: Female.
Approximate age: Early 60s.
Background information: The patient had suffered from rheumatism for many years. Treatment principally through a change of diet and the addition of herbal remedies had alleviated the condition. There were residual problems including a very severe continuous pain in the lumbar region causing much loss of sleep.
Condition treated: Rheumatism of the gluteal area.
Specific oils used: Basil on the lumbar gluteal area and No. 2 oil on the front to help the patient relax.
Frequency of treatment: A course of ten sessions spread over several weeks.
Result: After the third treatment the pain disappeared and the patient was able to sleep comfortably at night pain-free.
Comment: At the time of making this report there has been no return of the trouble.

★   ★   ★

Therapist: Hubert Lam, Canada.
Sex of patient: Female.
Approximate age: 45.
Background information: Had received various other forms of treatment over a number of years but with no lasting effect.
Condition treated: Muscle spasms in back combined with nervous tension.
Oils used: Geranium and No. 2.
Frequency of treatment: Once a month.
Result: Great improvement both physically and psychologically.

★   ★   ★

Therapist: Iris Rigazzi-Tarling, Chertsey, Surrey.
Sex of patient: Female.
Approximate age: 50.
Background information: Not available.
Condition treated: Severe blow to elbow, stiffening of joint, considerable swelling of area.
Oil used: Basil.
Frequency of treatment: Twice.
Result: Swelling subsided, joint became easily moveable and after the second treatment no further pain was experienced and the swelling had gone completely.

Comment: The therapist involved records that the situation was a completely spontaneous one, having met the patient a short while after the accident happened. Basil was the only oil she had with her at the time.

★   ★   ★

Therapist: Sandy Hemingway, London.
Sex of patient: Male.
Approximate age: Late 50s.
Background information: The patient was a plumber who felt that his condition resulted from occupational hazards because he had to keep his neck and head in such odd positions. He had suffered from very bad headaches for a long time and claimed that he had not slept through the night for at least six years.
Condition treated: Rheumatism of the shoulders and neck.
Specific oils used: Sage for the neck and basil on the head and forehead.
Frequency of treatment: Three times in total.
Result: The head which had been locked in a forward position moved easily and the headaches disappeared.
Comment from the patient: He said that his head now felt as though it had been oiled as it moved so easily and he had slept like a baby.

★   ★   ★

Therapist: Anne Ward, Surfers Paradise, Australia.
Sex of patient: Female.
Approximate age: 40.
Background information: Patient exhibited a well balanced attitude to life, complained of having a tired back and painful right leg since childhood, yet had a good vertical though rather stiff posture. She had received physiotherapy, chiropractic and osteopathic treatment all with moderate but only temporary success.
Condition treated: Scoliosis in back and muscular tension in leg.
Oils used: Jasmin, rosemary and lemongrass.
Frequency of treatment: Once a week.
Result: The scoliosis which was quite clear on the X-ray photographs but was obviously of psychosomatic origin cleared up as did the trouble in the leg, neither of which have re-appeared.

Chapter 14

Neurological Case Histories

Therapist: Valerie Anne Worwood, Romford, Essex.
Sex of patient: Female.
Approximate age: 55.
Background information: The client was widowed at an early age and left to bring up three children. Has suffered from migraine since childhood, recently getting very depressed and anxious.
Condition treated: Migraine and depression.
Principal oil used: Lavender.
Frequency of treatment: Once a week for six weeks.
Result: Only one migraine occured during the course of treatment. Patient now has headaches very infrequently, all tension in the neck has been eased.
Comment: The patient had received a variety of medical treatments over a period of years with no positive results.

✶   ✶   ✶

Therapist: Sandy M. Hemingway, London.
Sex of patient: Male.
Approximate age: 30.
Background information: A history of the same disease in the patient's family. The young man concerned has received medical treatment over a long period but the disease condition had still progressed.
Condition treated: Multiple sclerosis.
Oils used (but not necessarily all at the same time):   Lemongrass to the front of the legs to tone muscles and tendons and geranium at the back to invigorate blood circulation, rosemary in the gluteal area and No. 2 oil and basil on the whole of the back but particularly the spinal area to which special attention was paid.

Frequency of treatments: A series of ten treatments at intervals of 6 to 7 days. After a 4 months occupational absence from home he now endeavours to have treatment about once a week.

Result: At commencement of treatment his symptoms were mainly in pelvic leg area which were accompanied by attacks of numbness making it extremely difficult to move the legs at all. After periods of standing his legs would fail to support him. He was very pale, extremely tense and said he had been sleeping badly. At the end of the first treatment, the patient said his body felt lighter and relaxed and he was even a little sleepy. The following day he reported that in the evening of the treatment he had felt very invigorated and relaxed and had slept very well for the first time in months. During the treatment his general health greatly improved, he achieved a good colour and resumed such athletic activities as tennis. The attacks of numbness in the pelvic leg area became infrequent.

Comment: At the time of this report it is 8 months since the client first reported for treatment and the improvement in his condition has continued.

Comment by the Author: It is well known in multiple sclerosis that there are periods at which the patient is better than at others (known as remission). However, these are usually much shorter periods than in the case quoted above and here there is no evidence of the worsening of the condition as one would expect. However, the author would caution against treating this as a cure but rather an improvement in the condition. In his opinion a treatment which improves mobility, reduces tension, improves sleep and enables the patient to resume normal activities must be considered a very great help in the treatment of such a difficult disease.

Herpes Simplex: Since his teens the author has been troubled with herpes simplex (cold sores on his upper lip). These appear with great regularity 4 to 5 times a year. A few years ago when he felt one coming, he massaged the area well with basil and the sore did not develop. Since then whenever the increased tenderness of the upper lip indicated a sore developing, he has applied the same basil treatment and has not now suffered a cold sore for several years.

Chapter 15

Vascular Case Histories

Therapist: Sandy M. Hemingway, London.
Sex of patient: Female.
Approximate age: 60.
Background of patient: A music teacher.
Condition treated: Patient requested a general relaxation massage.
Specific oils used: Sage for the back and jasmin for the front with geranium on the legs as there was some indication of poor circulation.
Result: At the time of this report she is a new patient and has only received one treatment. The patient reported by letter a few days later that she felt wonderful and friends had commented on the improvement of her facial colour. In the letter she revealed that she had for a long time suffered from blood pressure which had remained fairly steady at 168/105. She was amazed to find the day after the treatment this had dropped to 120/70.
Comment by the therapist: I was very surprised at the contents of the letter because the patient had not revealed or indicated in any way this blood pressure problem. This made the results particularly gratifying to me.

★   ★   ★

Therapist: Wanda Simenacz, Croydon, Surrey.
Sex of patient: Female.
Approximate age: Over 70.
Condition treated: Pain and discomfort arising from varicose veins.
Oil used: Geranium.
Frequency of treatment: A few treatments in the clinic then daily home treatments by the patient herself.
Result: Considerable relief from pain; tiredness and discomfort disappearing.
Comment: The patient comments that she feels the regular home treatment is now essential for her because of the relief that it has brought.

Chapter 16

Skin and Face Case Histories

Therapist: Valerie Ann Worwood, Romford, Essex.
Sex of patient: Male.
Approximate age: 36.
Background information: The patient is a professional singer very well known throughout the world and has had many hit records and is also a successful song writer. Financially very secure and with a happy marriage. On the surface the patient is very calm and this is how he appears although inside is very nervous and tense.
Condition treated: Rapidly ageing and dehydrated skin combined with a sinus problem causing him a great deal of distress because of his work. This increased his tension.
Oils used: Sandalwood, lavender and jasmin.
Frequency of treatment: Twice a week for three weeks. In between treatments the patient used the same oils at home. The intensity of treatment being necessary because of patient's working engagements.
Result: The patient's skin became more pliable, all the flakiness had stopped and he looked 5 years younger. He was also much more relaxed.
Comment by therapist: Since the treatment the patient has felt very good in himself, his sinus problem has been much easier and he has been in better voice than for a long time.

The above therapist records the following history.
Sex of patient: Female.
Approximate age: 33.
Background information: A housewife with a working class background. Lost her husband several years ago and was left to bring up three children. Has financial and emotional problems caused in part by the children growing up. The patient

75

has a medical history of several reproductive problems and increasingly depressed state of mind due to a worsening acne problem and dilated pores which resemble scarring of the skin.

Condition treated: Acne.

Oils used: Lavender and lemongrass alternatively.

Frequency of treatment: Once a week for three weeks with the client using the oil at home in between.

Result: After first treatment the condition started to clear up within 3 days. By the end of the first week the pustules had completely disappeared and the dilated pores looked a lot better.

Comment by the therapist: Not only did the patient look very much better, but she reported that she had been able to cope much more easily with conditions at home and is now continuing a home treatment with lemongrass to complete closure of the pores.

★   ★   ★

Therapist: Beryl M. Bell, Nottingham.

Sex of patient: Female.

Approximate age: 27.

Background history: Not available.

Condition treated: Extreme external seborrhoea.

Oil used: Ylang-ylang.

Frequency of treatment: Once a week.

Result: Seborrhoea completely cleared.

Comment: In addition to the clearing of the seborrhoea the patient has become very relaxed.

★   ★   ★

Therapist: Eileen Lazar, Sydney, Australia.

Sex of patient: Female.

Approximate age: Not given.

Background information: A technical college lecturer, heavy in build, her facial skin completely lifeless. The overall picture was of a very exhausted person who completely lacked interest in herself.

Oils used: Sage and sandalwood on the body, ylang-ylang on the face combined with geranium cactus jelly mask.

Frequency of treatment: Continuing.

Result: At the end of the first treatment her skin glowed, she exhibited more self interest and a feeling of wellbeing.

Comment: The patient was so pleased with the result of her treatment she took the trouble to come to the clinic the following day to say how wonderful she felt.

The above therapist reports a similar case history of a small lady who had very white lifeless skin, holds a very responsible secretarial position and who was referred by a local doctor. In this case the patient also suffered from rheumatism so she received body treatment as well as facial treatment. Neroli cream and cactus jelly mask were used on the face with sage and lemongrass on the body. The therapist reports in this case that not only has the patient's skin improved considerably and the rheumatism improved but the patient herself is enjoying work and life very much more since she started the treatment.

★   ★   ★

Therapist: Irene Latter, Glasgow.
Sex of patient: Female.
Approximate age: 30.
Condition treated: Boil type eruption proximal thigh inner aspect.
Oil used: Basil.
Frequency of treatment: Once in the clinic and daily at home with the same oil.
Result: The patient phoned the following day saying the swelling had reduced by half and the nagging drawing pain had gone. By the fourth day it had completely disappeared.
Comment: The patient was advised to report to her own doctor as a precaution. It is doubtful whether she did because this very worried lady had now become so happy.

★   ★   ★

Therapist: Marjorie E. Marris, Staines.
Sex of patient: Female.
Approximate age: 52.
Background information: Wife of businessman, is overweight and overactive.
Condition treated: Psoriasis mainly on hands and arms and hyperactivity.
Oils used: Lavender, sandalwood and jasmin.
Frequency of treatment: Once a month for three months, but treatment supplemented with same oils applied at home 2 or 3 times a week. Patient was also advised to use Bain d'Aromes in her bath most evenings before retiring.
Result: The psoriasis has completely disappeared and the patient is much more relaxed.
Comment: Mrs. Marris says that this patient suffered from psoriasis for a number of years and is absolutely delighted with the result. Mrs. Marris was herself a sufferer from psoriasis

which was so severe that it was not possible to place a finger between the lesions on her leg. She treated herself in the way described above and it was the complete clearing of the condition which encouraged her to use it on other patients.

★   ★   ★

Therapist: Petra Zuidema, St. Albert, Alberta, Canada.
Sex of patient: Female.
Approximate age: 35.
Background information: Client was a public health nurse.
Condition treated: Acne.
Oils used: Formula No. 1, tangerine, lavender and lemongrass.
Frequency of treatment: Once a week for eight weeks, then every ten days totalling in all 5 months.
Result: The condition has completely cleared and there is no visible scarring.
Comment: Client had suffered from this condition for a number of years and is now more than happy with her beautiful skin.

★   ★   ★

Therapist: Wanda Simenacz, Croydon, Surrey.
Sex of patient: Female.
Approximate age: 16.
Condition treated: Severe acne rosacea.
Oil used: Ylang-ylang.
Frequency of treatment: Three treatments in 2 months.
Result: A spectacular clearing of the condition.
Comment: The patient came not expecting any improvement but was so delighted with the result that she recommended two of her acquaintances with similar conditions.

The above therapist also reports:
Sex of patient: Female.
Approximate age: 40.
Background information: Client is a medical doctor.
Condition treated: Tired, neglected facial skin.
Oil used: Lavender.
Frequency of treatment: Once a month.
Result: Complete rejuvenation of the face, the skin having recovered its freshness and elasticity.

The above therapist also reports:

Sex of patient: Female.

Approximate age: 40.

Background information: Wife of a medical consultant with hospital appointment.

Condition treated: Facial skin in very poor condition.

Oils used: Lavender and sandalwood.

Frequency of treatment: Regular monthly treatments.

Result: Marked improvement in the skin with increased elasticity and a new freshness of aspect.

Comment: Her housekeeper was so impressed with the results she now wishes to undertake similar treatment.

The above therapist also reports:

Sex of patient: Female.

Approximate age: 25.

Background information: Client is a nurse.

Condition treated: Extensive broken capillaries.

Oil used: Sandalwood.

Frequency of treatment: Monthly for approximately one year.

Result: Very marked improvement.

Chapter 17

Stress and Nervous Tension Case Histories

Therapist: Ernest Oliver Crouch, Hilton, Natal, South Africa.
Sex of patient: Female.
Approximate age: 48.
Background information: Married with one child, well educated, lives to a hectic schedule which includes a great deal of social work. Tends to overdo things, falls back on drugs to stabilise and stimulate herself. This situation has continued over a period of years and it was observed that in addition to the condition treated the patient suffered from spastic colon, varicose veins and much bruising on the legs.
Condition treated: Constant state of nervous tension.
Oils used: Sandalwood, sage and No. 2.
Frequency of treatment: Once a month for a period of five months.
Result: Restored both physically and mentally, able to cope with her day to day chores.
Comment by therapist: The infrequency of the treatment only emphasises the efficiency of the techniques used and the healing powers of the natural oils.

★   ★   ★

Therapist: Anne Roebuck, Toronto, Canada.
Sex of patient: Female.
Approximate age: 42.
Background information: Vice-president of a T.V. commercial company, divorced supporting two children. Presented for treatment after having worked for three weeks non-stop shooting a series of T.V. commercials for a large

corporation, had not slept properly for over a month, totally exhausted physically and mentally. Unable at this stage to continue her professional career due to exhaustion.

Condition treated: Insomnia, nervous and physical exhaustion which involved mild cystitis.

Principal oils used: Basil, geranium and sandalwood.

Frequency of treatment: Every day for 4 days and 1 further treatment 3 days later.

Result: Rapid recovery, sleeping 7½ hours a night, no cystitis, full of energy and 1 week after commencing treatment able to fly off to another field location which she would have had to cancel and lose to a big competitor.

The above therapist also reports the following case:

Sex of patient: Female.

Approximate age: 59.

Background information: A department store sales lady who had received open heart surgery 2 months previously. Miss Roebuck consulted the patient's cardiologist before commencing treatment and his permission was given with enthusiasm.

Condition treated: Very stiff neck and shoulders because the patient had to sleep on her back propped up with pillows after surgery and full of tension after the shock of surgery.

Oil used: No. 2.

Frequency of treatment: Three times a week for two weeks.

Result: The muscle stiffness disappeared completely and the patient was very much more relaxed.

Chapter 18

Miscellaneous Case Histories

Therapist: R. W. Carter, Chelmsford.
Sex of patient: Female.
Approximate age: 40.
Background information: Highly strung, energetic, a retail products promoter.
Condition treated: Sinusitis.
Oil used: Geranium.
Frequency of treatment: Monthly but supported by regular application at home of the same oil.
Result: Sinusitis condition cleared up quickly.
Comment: Patient reported the success of the treatment to her doctor who appeared to be suitably impressed.

★   ★   ★

Therapist: Eileen Lazar, Sydney, Australia.
Sex of patient: Female.
Approximate age: 40.
Background information: Married with three teenage children, husband a busy executive, she has part-time employment in a boutique. Very nervous and irritable, always complaining, yet has everything that she could wish for.
Condition treated: Cellulitis and aches and pains brought on through nervous tension.
Oils used: Basil and sage on the body, lavender alternating with jasmin on the face.
Frequency of treatment: Initially weekly then fortnightly.
Result: Excellent.
Comment by therapist: 'At first I was a physical wreck after treating her but now she is so gentle with me that I look forward to her visits.'

Therapist: Valerie Ann Worwood, Romford, Essex.
Sex of patient: Female.
Approximate age: 32.
Background information: Client is a wealthy woman with no particular medical or marital problem but is generally rundown and bored. She had started to reorganise her body, has had a breast operation and was thinking of having her buttocks reduced by cosmetic surgery.
Condition treated: Nothing in particular – client thought she'd like to try it!
Oils used: Jasmin and geranium.
Frequency of treatment: Once a week for six weeks.
Result: These were surprising, scar tissue which she still had from the breast operation had diminished to become almost invisible. She started to get interested in her husband's career and was thinking of doing something herself. She gained confidence in her appearance and decided not to have her buttocks reduced.

★　　★　　★

Therapist: Bernice Davis, (Kristine Faith), Scotland.
Sex of patient: Male.
Approximate age: 10.
Background information: Since a baby this child has been allergic to eggs in any form.
Condition treated: Accidental burn to the arm.
Oil used: Special formula No. 2.
Result: Excellent.
Comment: Whilst on holiday on the Greek Island of Rhodes a waiter in the hotel accidentally spilt boiling hot coffee over the young boy's arm. He was immediately rushed into the kitchen by the staff for first aid. The Greek first aid treatment for burns is to cover the area with the white of eggs – not knowing of course that the boy was allergic to eggs this was done. By the time he was returned to his mother (Mrs. Davis) his arm was very red, swollen and painful. Mrs. Davis rushed him to her room where the only essential oil she had was No. 2 which she used herself. She quickly completely covered the area with this oil and within a very short period of time the child's arm was perfectly healed with no blistering or scarring.

★　　★　　★

Therapist: Anne Ward, Surfers Paradise, Australia.
Sex of patient: Female.
Approximate age: 22.
Background information: Ex-trainee nurse for two years then gave up with no occupation since. The emaciation part of her condition having been caused by living in poor conditions in the East.
Condition treated: Emaciation, tiredness, out of touch with reality but with a supressed anger, she simply sat and stared without blinking, uncooperative, non-speaking, rigid, limbs held closely to the body.
Oils used: Geranium, ylang-ylang and jasmin.
Frequency of treatment: Twice a week.
Result: The rigid, vertebral column has relaxed, the client looks better, feels better and smiles.
Comment by therapist: Gradually the essential oils restored life to this lass; like a miracle unfolding seeing her progress at the end of each treatment, towards reintegrating with the human race. She was gradually feeling life flowing back into her body.

Chapter 19

Epilogue

The case histories recorded in Part II were supplied in response to a questionnaire sent by the writer to some of his former students. He would like to thank them for being so co-operative and to say that space limitations prevent the inclusion of all the histories they sent in. He would also like to thank Patricia Lam, Toronto, Canada, Sally McMeekin, Theydon Bois, Essex and Susanne Saville, Farnham, who also responded but whose replies it was not possible to include principally because they were near duplicates of other cases already quoted or because they arrived after the main scripts had gone to the printers.

To the above and all serious practitioners of this therapy, may your patients long continue to enjoy the good health which essential oils are helping to make possible. It is not claimed as being a panacea for all ills but rather as one of the very practical aids to the healthy enjoyment of life.

Appendix

PRODUCTS

Most of the oils are to Madame Marguerite Maury's original formulae.

In the United Kingdom the facial strength oils are sold in 50ml amber bottles and the body strength oils in 100ml amber bottles.

Bath oils are packaged in 15ml dropper bottles and the cactus jelly masks and Neroli creams are packaged in the United Kingdom in 100g jars.

Basil	Sage
Eucalyptus	Sandalwood
Geranium	Tangerine
Jasmin	Thyme
Lavender	Ylang-ylang
Lemongrass	Formula No. 1
Neroli	Formula No. 2
Peppermint	Formula No. 3
Rosemary	

Neroli Cream when used in beauty treatments is a night cream suitable for all ages except those persons with very oily skins: used in the field of therapy, it is valuable in reducing the risk of scarring after burns and is a good treatment for bruises as well as helping to reduce swelling.

Neroli Arome is a day cream when used in beauty therapy and additional foundation is not necessary. In the field of therapy, it may be used for the same purposes as Neroli Cream but where a non oily substance is desired.

Cactus jelly masks – Geranium, Lavender, Sandalwood and Jasmin.

Bath oils – for an average size domestic bath, about 5–10 drops are needed. Added to the bath water under the hot tap whilst the bath is being filled.

Bain de Jouvence has a very invigorating, rejuvenating and stimulating effect.

Bain d'Aromes reduces body tension, relaxes muscles with a good physiological effect, intended as a bedtime bath oil.

Aromatherapy Milk supplied in ½ litre containers.

A current price list on the products may be obtained on application to Mrs Kim Aldridge, Oakelbrook Mill, Newent, Gloucestershire GL18 1HD.

TRAINING

Training seminars for Aromatherapy Diploma and Phys-essential Therapy Diploma are regularly held in the United Kingdom, as well as Europe, and many other parts of the world. Such training is only available to persons who are already qualified or are in the final stages of their professional training and may be undertaken by members of all the para-medical professions as well as beauty therapists. Interested persons are invited to apply to Arnould-Taylor Education, James House, Oakelbrook Mill, Newent, Glos., GL18 1HD, telephone 0531 821875, who will be pleased to send full details of such courses, their dates, venue, cost and duration. It should be emphasised that the training courses have a high content of practical work. Theoretical knowledge is not sufficient, practical skills have also to be acquired.

EQUIPMENT

Brochures and prices of equipment mentioned in this book may be obtained from the George Solly Organisation Limited, 111 Watlington Street, Reading, Berks RG1 4RQ. Telephone: 0734 566 477. Fax: 0734 566 318.